Down Syndrome

Human Potentials for Children Series

Down Syndrome:
Growing and Learning

Siegfried M. Pueschel
Claire D. Canning
Ann Murphy
Elizabeth Zausmer

Down Syndrome

Growing and Learning

Edited by
Siegfried M. Pueschel, M.D., M.P.H.

Andrews, McMeel & Parker
A Universal Press Syndicate Company
Kansas City ● New York

First printing, September 1978
Sixth printing, January 1986

Library of Congress Cataloging in Publication Data
Main entry under title:
Down syndrome.
    (Human potentials for children series)
Bibliography: p.
    1. Down's syndrome. 2. Mentally handicapped
children—Care and treatment. 3.Mentally handicapped
children—Rehabilitation. I. Pueschel, S. M.
II. Series.
RJ506.D68D68   362.7'8'3   78-19184
ISBN 0-8362-2804-9
ISBN 0-8362-2805-7 pbk.

To
CHRIS AND MARTHA

Contents

Bibliography

Foreword

This is not a book about a syndrome but a book about children. These children have some chromosomes which happen to be arranged in special ways, and the arrangement is referred to as Down Syndrome. If the emphasis is on the syndrome, it may appear that the children are much alike, and constitute a clearly defined "category." But if the syndrome is pushed into the background, if the children are liberated from being chained to this category and are looked at as individuals, it will be clear that they differ quite markedly one from another, that indeed they are more similar to the average child in the community than they are different in the ways they grow and develop.

When we read this book we thought of the many families we have come to know in different countries who have a child born with Down Syndrome. How much their lives would have been enriched, how much their child's physical and social well-being would have improved if only they had had access to the information Dr. Pueschel and his coauthors offer in this volume. But it is of course not just a matter of information; on every page there is reflected an attitude of respect and warmth of feeling toward handicapped children, and in particular, those with Down Syndrome who for so long have been labeled and libeled as ineducable and incompetent. As "Mongoloids" they have been subjected to stereotyping and prejudicial downgrading even by those who are proud of their lack of prejudice when it comes to racial and religious differences. The "self-fulfilling prophecy" of their supposed deficiencies kept them excluded from many helpful programs and activities.

In contrast to the unhappy frustrations of the past, *Down Syndrome: Growing and Learning* provides the families, the professional workers and the volunteers with detailed, readily understood guidance to further the physical, social, mental, and emotional development of the child with Down Syndrome, giving particular emphasis to earliest intervention. For the professional worker as well as for the family, the teamwork that produced this book will have more than symbolic meaning, it demonstrates that success will depend on positive interaction between them all.

Gunnar Dybwad, M.D.
and Rosemary Dybwad, M.D.

Acknowledgments

The authors are foremost indebted to the many wonderful children with Down Syndrome and their extraordinary parents, for without their cooperation and contributions, this book would never have been written. Both parents and their children taught us so much so that we in turn may teach others.

We also would like to express our gratitude to the many professionals who participated in the Down Syndrome Program at the Developmental Evaluation Clinic of Children's Hospital Medical Center: the nurses, Susan Cullen, Marie Cullinane, and Eunice Shishmanian; the physicians, Allen C. Crocker, Liza Yessayan, and Margaret Siber; the psychologists, Richard Schnell, Patricia Boyle, and Betsy Kammerer; the anthropologists, Mary Ann Whelan and Christine Cronk; the physical therapists, Alice Shea, Diana Nathan, and Joanne Valvano; the nutritionists, Rosanne Howard and Carol Hum; and the many other coworkers in the Developmental Evaluation Clinic and the Hearing and Speech Department of Children's Hospital Medical Center who were at one time or another involved in the Down Syndrome Program. We thank the able coordinators who have been with the program over the past years: Diane Barendse, Linda Duchak, and Anita Wilson.

In particular, we would like to express our appreciation to Allen C. Crocker, Director of the Developmental Evaluation Clinic, for the guidance, advice and support he provided to the program. We wish to thank Jean Zadig,

William Kiernan, Otto Zausmer, and Harriet Klebanoff for their review of the manuscript and their valuable comments. We are most grateful to Dr. Gunnar Dybwad for his thorough critique and his outstanding suggestions. We would like to acknowledge the excellent editorial work by Will Lehr who spent so much time in improving the text of this book.

We are indebted to Joseph Canning and Linda Duchack for their photographic skills which brought life to many chapters of this book. Dr. Renee Vogel kindly provided us with photographs of chromosomes including a metaphase and various karyotypes. We especially would like to thank Linda Crepeau and JoAnne Meehan for their secretarial assistance.

Part of the work of the Down Syndrome Program was supported by MCHS Project 928 and by NICHD Grant HDO 5341-03, U.S. Department of Health, Education, and Welfare.

Introduction

During the past two decades considerable progress in the biomedical and behavioral sciences has brought forth new and more effective approaches in the care and education of handicapped individuals. Concurrently, a greater awareness and determination led parents of retarded youngsters to secure for their children the rights and opportunities available to other children. These developments in turn have gradually fostered attitudinal changes in society including a greater acceptance of developmentally disabled persons.

As the authors of this book we have actively participated in these evolutionary processes as professionals, parents, and members of society. Three of us have had the opportunity to work at the Developmental Evaluation Clinic of the Children's Hospital Medical Center in Boston for the past ten years. In 1970 we initiated—together with other professionals—an extensive study of children with Down Syndrome and since then we have followed closely the growth and development of several hundred children with Down Syndrome. This work allowed us to learn intimately of the parents' concerns, to investigate the children's developmental function and their needs, and how to best provide optimal stimulation and environmental enrichment to their lives.

Beyond such professional involvement two of us are parents who have a child with Down Syndrome. This personal experience in rearing a child with Down Syndrome and the fundamental encounter of sorrow and joy perhaps will add to this book, we believe, an extra dimension that is difficult to express by the professional worker who is less directly involved.

As members of society, the way we think and work, of course, has been influenced by attitudes prevalent in society. At the same time, we have also attempted to initiate changes by educating society and thus have altered and modified the less desirable attitudes toward handicapped persons.

The above mentioned profound experiences and involvements—in addition to others—provided the basic elements for the compilation of this book. Hence the book, *Down Syndrome: Growing and Learning,* is written from real life situations and it is intended to make the child's life a happier and more fulfilling one.

While we attempt to cover the entire lifespan of the person with Down Syndrome, we do not deal with every aspect of life in depth and detail. Rather, this book will give an overview, highlighting significant developmental periods and aspects in the life of the person with Down Syndrome. In addition, it focuses on important aspects of Down Syndrome as a handicapping condition.

This book is not intended as a textbook for students and professionals. It does not give a systematic description of specific medical, psychological, and educational issues on Down Syndrome for instructional purposes. While our primary aim is to provide updated information to parents who have a child with Down Syndrome, many professionals undoubtedly will also find certain chapters of this book useful and educational. Whether they be parents, siblings, or other interested individuals, readers will gain a deeper understanding of the subject of Down Syndrome.

We hope that readers will share the basic philosophy we express in this book and that improvement in the quality of all aspects of life of the person with Down Syndrome will soon become a societal reality.

=1

FROM PARENT
TO PARENT

Claire D. Canning

Of all the joys and sorrows of a lifetime of living, no event in our lives was ever more traumatic than the birth of Martha, our daughter with Down Syndrome. We were shocked, shattered, bewildered. No one really ever expects to give birth to a defective child. Prior to Martha's birth, mental retardation had been simply a statistic to us, something that inevitably happens to someone else. Yet, in five short years, Martha has taught us so much.

If you are the parent of an older child with Down Syndrome, you are already aware of the very special bond that exists between parents who have shared the same intense sorrows and joys. If you are a professional, I beg you to keep pace with the progress being made in the field of mental retardation, and to take the time to see each child as a human being. If you are in the field of special education or a related field, know that your encouragement and reinforcement can add invaluable dimensions to the life of the mentally retarded child and his family.

If you are a new parent, I can share the deep sorrow you feel in every fiber of your being, the aching disappointment, the hurt pride, the terrible fear of the unknown; but I can tell you from personal experience that having known this ultimate sorrow, you will soon learn to cope better with every phase of life. You will be happy once again, and through your child you will receive undreamed of love, joy, and satisfaction.

Life cannot remain the same: the decision to choose a profession, a new career, the choice to marry or to have a child—all important judgments in our life—imply change. The addition to a family of a child with Down Syndrome precipitates even more rapid change, but the loving support you will meet at each phase will be an enriching experience.

My first fear was for our marriage. If it had been a shaky commitment, the Down Syndrome child could have provided us with an opportunity to blame each other, or to make excuses for never finding time for self or others. But if you work at it, this special child can be the opportunity for better communication, for finding new courage and love in your partner. Personally, I have never appreciated my husband so much; the feeling of mutual support has enhanced our marriage.

I feared for our other children. I wanted to give them enough time so that they would not feel neglected or harbor unspoken feelings of shame or resentment. Their response, their potential for love, has overwhelmed us. They have given us courage in so many ways, and in turn they have not been cheated, but enriched. Together, we have all learned the dignity and worth of each human being.

I feared so for our new little child, Martha. This was surely not the life I had intended to give her. But I have learned that her little life is a very precious thing, that she is singularly happy, and loves unquestioningly with a degree that makes me wonder just what constitutes "normality." She has truly been a joy to us all.

Compared to the bleak future that awaited the mentally

retarded child of the past, this last decade has seen considerable progress for the child with special needs, perhaps more than the last sixty years which preceded it. The public in general seems to be experiencing a new compassion and awareness. Although as a parent you must work to pursue them, new programs and services are available—even mandated by law—to guide and support you.

After an initial period of trauma, we were very fortunate to find a marvelous program for Down Syndrome children run by professionals whose expertise and genuine love and respect for the dignity of every human being guided us through our most difficult days. Fortunately, similar programs in which human services and guidance aid you in planning for your child's development are now beginning to exist all over the country. The professionals in our program have been far more than advisors to us; they are friends to whom we will always be grateful.

One of the particular advantages we have experienced is the friendship of other parents, very beautiful people who have successfully combined their own careers with the loving care of special children. We would never have had the opportunity to know these friends without Martha. They have unflinchingly worked against what we once felt to be great odds. Their courage has inspired us and caused us to look more realistically at life's true values. Older friendships have become even richer as our friends seem to share a special pride in Martha's accomplishments. I like to think that the entire community has profited and their kindness and compassion are overwhelming.

As for Martha herself, how do I think of her today as a child of five? I am in constant awe of all she knows and understands. She is enrolled in a special class in an integrated public school where a beautiful learning atmosphere and a feeling of community support have amazed us. Pre-primary training at school, and constant stimulation at home, have been invaluable.

You will soon learn that the child with Down Syndrome does almost everything a normal child does, but more slowly. With love and understanding, these children can achieve many things heretofore unexpected of them. At five, Martha not only walks, she runs. She is fully toilet trained, is self-feeding, tries to dress herself, and hangs up her clothing. She bursts with independence, speaks in phrases, knows her colors, counts to ten, and to our utter amazement, can not only spell her own name but is actually beginning to read. She has a definite sense of humor, a great sense of the ridiculous, and learns a great deal from socialization and imitation. She loves music, travels well, and has a sensitive appreciation for the tiniest favor. She responds well to gentle discipline. I have come to think of her as a bundle of mischief, an imp with sticky fingers, and only incidentally, as a child with a handicap.

What do I wish for her in the future? I think the most valuable thing we can give Martha is complete acceptance of her just as she is, and a desire to make her as independent as possible for the future. From the community, I ask for compassion, but not pity, and a chance to prove herself as fully as possible with all the rights of a human being within her capabilities. Our greatest hope is that some day when we are no longer here, the institutions as we now know them will have been replaced by carefully supervised group homes within the community, where all people with Down Syndrome may live and know the joys of friendship, the dignity of self-worth, and the usefulness of work in a protected atmosphere.

As parents, we have learned that there is little more we

can wish for any of our children, but that each develop his potential to the best of his abilities. In the end, the material accomplishments of this world won't matter much at all. What will endure is the quality of love we have given to others. For us, what seemed like the tragedy of our lives has become our greatest and most fulfilling opportunity.

2

A CHILD
WITH DOWN SYNDROME
IS BORN

Ann Murphy

Learning That You Have a Handicapped Child

The birth of a child is a very important event in the life of any family. There are nine months to make practical arrangements regarding care, clothing, space, and furnishings. Simultaneously and more importantly, parents imagine what this new family member will be like. They will have dreams about what the newcomer may accomplish. During these nine months, most parents voice some concern that possibly something may go wrong, but this is usually fleeting and brushed aside, particularly if there have been no problems with the pregnancy and if there is no family member with a handicap.

Then the day finally arrives: you give birth. Will your expectations and your anticipations become true? You sense, you feel something is not quite right. You notice a tenseness and anxiety in the staff attending the delivery or in others involved in caring for you and the baby immediately afterward. The nurses do not seem very enthusiastic or excited. Your physician advises you that there are concerns about the baby's condition. Perhaps you yourself have noticed something different about the child's appearance or the way he feels when you hold him. You are afraid. Then you are informed by your doctor that your newborn child has Down Syndrome. The words are unfamiliar and mean little until you learn that this is the scientific term for what used to be known as "Mongolism."

All parents who have experienced this moment describe sensations of overwhelming shock and disbelief. It feels as though the world is coming to an end. It is hard to listen further to words and explanations which the doctor is offering because all your energies are absorbed in the feelings and images people have about mental retardation and Down Syndrome. You may remember some individuals who were obese, clumsy, unappealing. Even many educated and medically sophisticated people think that a retarded child looks different, that his head may be large and misshapen, that he does not have the potential to react like others, that he cannot recognize family members or respond to them with love and affection. Most parents express fear and the desire "to be out of the situation."

"I was like a little kid. I wanted to say take it away, take it back, but I knew it wouldn't go away."

"I wished the child was dead, deaf, blind, anything but retarded."

Some people try to escape the overwhelming reality by hoping some mistake has been made, that the chromosome test will prove the doctor wrong, that their child will be an exception. Many parents are concerned that there is something wrong with them if such things come up in their minds. However, these are very natural reactions to a crisis. They are expressions of the need of all human beings to try and escape what seems to be an untenable situation.

Even though you may be told that Down Syndrome

occurs once in every six to seven hundred births, you cannot help brood about why it happened to you. Most people search for an explanation within their own personal behavior or those close to them. They search for something that happened, something that was overlooked. They may blame themselves or others. It is sometimes easier blaming a person or a specific object for one's painful feelings rather than relating them to statistical abstractions. Many parents are fearful that having such a child reflects on their competence in some way and that other people may think less of them if they have given birth to a retarded child.

People handle their feelings in different ways: some by withdrawal into themselves, others in expressing their feelings openly—by crying or getting angry. Some people actively seek information, ask questions and make telephone calls, while others wait for people around them to volunteer their reactions and ideas. For most people it takes months before they regain a sense of their usual self, to get in touch with their normal routines and attachments. The feelings of sadness and loss never completely go away, but as a result of this experience many people describe a new perspective and sensitivity to what is truly important in life. Sometimes a shattering experience such as this can serve to strengthen and unify a family.

Getting to Know the Baby

Many parents acknowledge a reluctance to get close to the baby. Some are afraid to look because they fear the baby may have an odd or unusual appearance. Others are timid about having physical contact with the child. They feel that somehow by touching, they are claiming the child as their own and committing themselves to assuming responsibility for his future. There are parents who are uncertain about accepting a child with a disability into their family life, investing their feelings in a person who may bring sadness rather than pleasure. Once the parents overcome their inhibitions and actually begin to look at the child, touch him, hold him, and care for him, they are often impressed with the fact that he is, after all, a baby and in most ways resembles other babies more than he is different from them. The opportunity to have contact with the child can enhance the feeling of normalcy. As with any new baby, most parental energy is channeled into learning his individual characteristics. Parents may soon be so impressed with his normal appearance and behavior that they find it hard to believe there is anything wrong. They find it hard to reconcile his relatively normal appearance and behavior with the serious implications of the diagnosis. Some parents describe endless hours inspecting and observing the baby, trying to capture his "differentness." The period of time involved in becoming reasonably comfortable with the child varies from family to family. On hearing the diagnosis some parents experience a very strong protective urge. Others continue to be uncertain and unsure about their feelings for months. A few are really unable to relate to a child with a handicap. One parent described the process in the following way: "First I realized what she would never be, then I learned what she did not have to be, and finally I think I have come to terms with what she is and can be." Such feelings of sadness and loss are apt to be revived when parents are feeling down or when there are reminders of what normal children can do and be that this child cannot.

Learning about Down Syndrome

Most parents need a considerable period of time, often

weeks and months, to organize in their minds what this child will be like, whether they can love him as they feel parents should, whether they will be able to provide him with the special care he may require. They try to envision what a future with him will be like, what problems will emerge, and how they might cope in the years to come. They try to compress all of the future into the present because they have no guidelines to draw upon to give them security in this new relationship and in making decisions about it. They need opportunities to express their feelings, ask questions, and have access to accurate information.

Unfortunately the professional staffs in many maternity hospitals are grappling with the same feelings and concerns that parents have. Their work allows them little contact with handicapped children, current philosophies, or new programs. Often their ideas are conditioned by their own previous experiences rather than factual knowledge and information. Sometimes they feel they should protect the parents by discouraging contact with the baby, which only serves to reinforce the parents' insecurity about getting to know the baby. They may even suggest that the child be placed away from home, not being aware that research has long demonstrated that the child's development will be adversely affected by growing up in an institution. Such a plan is also often detrimental to family adjustment because the decision to place the child in a residential facility at such an early period may be based on unfounded fears rather than on direct experience in caring for the child. Some doctors feel uncomfortable and pessimistic about retarded children because they have no specific cure they can offer to the family. They may have been improperly taught in medical school that the best place for such children is a residential facility. Physicians may sometimes be unaware of how much can be accomplished through education and training and that there are programs available for retarded children of all ages in most communities. Many doctors, of course, show empathy and understanding and offer support and guidance to families with Down Syndrome children.

Informing Other People

Once parents are convinced their child has Down Syndrome, they are often unsure whether to tell other people or what the appropriate timing is for doing so. Some families question whether it might not be better to keep it a secret until they have become more used to it themselves. Others feel that if other people know, it might prevent them from treating the child in a relaxed and normal way. However, most people will notice that there is something different about the child's appearance or else be aware of your tension and sadness. They usually will not initiate a conversation regarding your baby. The result may be awkwardness in relationships with close relatives and friends.

The desire to postpone informing these people may be an indication that you have not really accepted your child's handicap yourself. Talking about it makes it more real. Yet, it brings back the feelings you had when you first heard of the "misfortune." It reopens the wound, and in some ways it is a confirmation that what happened is real rather than a dream. Although painful, talking with other people about your child with Down Syndrome can be an important step in working through your own sadness and shock, in regaining your former confidence and personal equilibrium.

Often relatives and friends are uncertain about what

role they should play when they hear that the baby has a disability. They are fearful that their overtures will be interpreted as either an intrusion or a curiosity. They will welcome some clue that their presence is desired and that their support and interest will be helpful. Sometimes communications break down when parents are waiting for some proof that people close to them still care. It is usually wise to proceed with the usual routine followed by your hospital and community after the birth of the baby, such as having the child's picture taken and listing the birth in the community newspaper. These are activities you ordinarily would have planned, and they will help you to feel more like your usual self.

Talking with Your Other Children

Most parents are uncertain about what they should say to their other children. It is natural to want to protect them from the worries of adults. You may also be embarrassed to talk with them or feel guilty that somehow you have compromised their future by giving them a retarded sister or brother. Some parents underestimate the sensitivity of their children's feelings or their ability to note differences in the baby's appearance and developmental course. Experience has shown that it is important to talk with your other children soon after you have heard of your child's problem yourself.

Young children will sense your mood and they will note that you go to the doctor more often with the baby than you did with them. They will probably not be aware of the actual differences in the baby until they notice that he does not walk as soon as the brother or sister of a friend. Older children will note differences in appearance, as will their friends. When they are asked about it, they will feel more comfortable if they have information and an explanation to offer. They will also be interested in knowing what caused it and what can be done "to fix it." Adolescents may be more concerned about whether they will be more likely than the average person to reproduce a handicapped child. All ages can gain something by visiting the program or pediatrician to whom you take the child. The younger children can benefit by not feeling left out as well as by being part of such an activity. School age children and adolescents may have questions they want to discuss with professionals. They should be encouraged to ask questions, and some time should be set aside for this purpose. Some centers have programs specifically for the purpose of informing brothers and sisters of handicapped children.

3

RESOURCES FOR REARING A HANDICAPPED CHILD

Ann Murphy

Current social trends are increasingly supportive of families who are rearing handicapped children within the home. The objective is first of all to provide the range of resources and opportunities that were formerly only available to the normal child but at the same time provide supplementary assistance to alleviate some of the additional demands the handicapped child's care places on the family. Much of this progress has been made because of the initiative of individual parents and parent groups who organized and advocated for the rights of their children. Most large communities have organizations of parents who provide information about local resources available to retarded persons through publications and individual consultation. They often have regularly scheduled meetings as well as a variety of committees for study and action regarding the needs of handicapped and retarded children and their families. Sometimes they operate service programs, such as educational programs for preschool children, camping and recreational programs, as well as workshops for the training and occupation of adults. Parents, professionals, and other interested individuals are encouraged to participate. You can secure information about the existence of such programs and organizations in your community by writing to the Down's

Syndrome Congress, the National Association for Retarded Citizens, Closer-Look (a federally sponsored information service), or your state department of mental health and/or mental retardation.

Parents with handicapped children usually do not have access to the many sources of information available to parents of normal children. Friends and relatives are loath to comment and often are not knowledgeable regarding Down Syndrome. Yet, other parents of children with Down Syndrome can offer specific information as well as emotional support. Names of parents who may be available to help can be obtained through the local parents' organization, the maternity hospital, nurses, or your pediatrician. You might want to talk with more than one family because each person's experience and values are different. Do not be concerned about asking them direct questions or asking to see their child, since people who volunteer know how you feel because they have been through it. Any or all of these resources will provide some information. However, you should not allow other people to tell you how you should feel and exactly what is right for you. You will probably have a lot of questions about how you will cope with the future, which no one can answer for you. The most important thing is to get some idea about what the next few months may be like and to locate resources in your community. Getting books from a public library can be discouraging since collections are often outdated and based on statistics gathered on children who were placed in institutions. Consequently, be sure and note when the book was published and who wrote it.

An important source of support in rearing your child is the availability of a qualified pediatrician who is interested in the development of handicapped children.

Many pediatricians are more oriented toward the diagnosis and treatment of specific diseases and may feel unqualified to help you in assessing the developmental progress of the child. If so, he may be able to tell you more about what is wrong with your child than about what ways he is functioning well. You will certainly have plenty of opportunities to learn in what ways your child differs from other children, but if this is the principal focus of every visit with your pediatrician, such visits will not be of much assistance in helping you evaluate how you and your child are working together.

At times it may be difficult to identify your child's readiness to move on to more sophisticated methods of feeding or advanced developmental activities. These are questions that you can raise with your pediatrician if he has this kind of interest and preparation. Such a relationship can be very supportive to your personal morale. It is also important to locate a pediatric dentist who is skilled in working with handicapped children. He can advise you on the care of your child's teeth.

Furthermore, you may find help at a local teaching hospital that has a child development clinic. Such a facility is usually staffed with professionals from different disciplines who can offer a more comprehensive evaluation of your child. Also, their plan of care and management will focus on the total needs of your child.

Increasingly, we are finding that early, guided management of handicapped children may make a significant difference in their later functioning. There are many different opinions as to how and why it is helpful. Some people stress that the significant impact of early intervention programs is on the parents' morale since they offer parents a continuing relationship with someone who has a positive interest in their child. This in turn is thought to help them function more normally in their relationship with their child. Others stress that anticipatory guidance assists parents in identifying indicators of their child's readiness to move forward developmentally and provides technical knowledge which enhances the child's potential to act on this readiness. Thus, there is a prevention of secondary handicaps. Some feel that this early guided stimulation brings the child more in contact with his surroundings and accelerates learning and achievements. No one claims that such programs will actually cure a disability, but most parents who have had this kind of support and encouragement feel it is of immeasurable value in rearing a handicapped child. The professionals who staff such programs are from a variety of disciplines. Many have a background in early childhood education or social work. Others have more technical knowledge, such as physical therapists, occupational therapists, and nurses. Often they work in teams and make contact with families through home visits or at local health centers. Sometimes they work with children and families in small groups. Such programs are often sponsored by the department of mental health, parents' associations, and community nursing programs.

The modern philosophy of normalization has greatly influenced educational and recreational programming for handicapped children. Increasingly, parents have a variety of available options from which to choose, the decision being based on the individual needs of the child.

School systems are required by Federal (PL 94-142) and state law to develop educational programs for preschool handicapped children, often as young as age three and sometimes from birth onward. However, there is frequently a significant gap between what educational laws say and what is actually implemented in terms of available programs. These lags represent apathy on the part of some school officials and/or lack of sufficient funding to provide the services to all the children who may need them. Often, it has been the initiative of the parents in pressing for change that has made the difference in translating paper philosophy and regulations to actual programs. Currently, many states mandate that public schools continue responsibility for the education of the handicapped child until he is twenty-one years of age, if he is profiting from the education. There may be a gradual deemphasis on academic subjects and increased time spent on skill development, which should actually begin early in life, useful for independent living or vocational placement. In addition, there are both privately sponsored and state-operated training programs for retarded citizens. Each may focus on students of certain levels of ability.

Many communities have organizaed social and group experiences for retarded children and similar recreational experiences for retarded adults. These may be sponsored by the public school, parents' associations, or the municipal park and recreation department. Organizations which specialize in recreation such as the Boy Scouts or the Y increasingly feel some responsibility to include the handicapped in their recreational programs. Many communities have special swimming programs for the handicapped, even providing individualized instruction.

The future for a retarded citizen can potentially include the range of options open to normal citizens. However, resources at present fall far short of needs. In the past there were two choices: one was that the retarded person lived with his parents until this was no longer feasible. The only alternative, except to people of wealth, was a state institution, where the quality of care was often very poor. The current trend is to phase out large institutions and develop a variety of small, supervised group-living situations where residents have the maximum decision-making role. These group residences may be tax supported, operated by foundations or parent groups, or may be proprietary. Whenever possible, residents lead a normal life routine, attending a daily work program that is located away from the living situation and using the recreational opportunities available in the general geographical area. Costs may be covered by tax funds, private donations, parent contributions, income generated by the work of residents, or tax-supported stipends which they receive if they are considered too disabled to be employed.

Parents often ask whether there are particular financial subsidies available to families rearing a handicapped child. For most families there are none, but low income families may be eligible for Supplemental Social Security income which is available through the Social Security Office. If a family falls within the income guidelines, the handicapped individual receives a stipend to assist with living expenses and, in addition, becomes eligible for Medicaid, which covers all medical expenses. Many communities have some resources to assist the family with the care of a handicapped child. Some towns provide part-time homemakers under some circumstances. Others provide temporary residential care (respite care) for the severely handicapped child during family vacation periods or at times of illness. Most communities have counseling services to help families who are experiencing unusual problems in relation to the care of their handicapped child. Family service and child welfare agencies can help families think through the implications of a child's care for the family. Occasionally, it may be appropriate to think of having your handicapped child live apart from the family for part of the time—a summer camp experience might be very appropriate. The kind of resource considered for such a placement depends on the child's needs, the family's wishes and resources, and what is available in the way of alternatives in the local area.

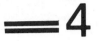

4

A HISTORICAL
VIEWPOINT

Siegfried M. Pueschel

Parents often wonder whether Down Syndrome has always been with mankind or whether it is a condition which only emerged in recent times. While there is no definitive answer to this question we assume that throughout biological history millions of evolutionary processes in the form of genetic changes and differentiations as well as chromosomal alterations must have occurred which would suggest that Down Syndrome is not an event of modern times.

Probably the earliest record stems from the excavation of a Saxon skull (seventh century) which is thought to be from a child with Down Syndrome because of the specific structural changes observed. There are also reports of some early paintings from the sixteenth and seventeenth centuries depicting children with features resembling Down Syndrome. Although it is assumed that these accounts convey that Down Syndrome has occurred in previous times there have not been any well documented reports of Down Syndrome prior to the nineteenth century. The reasons for this may be manifold: until recently there were only a limited number of medical journals available; there were only a few researchers interested in genetic problems; and other diseases such as infections and malnutrition were so prevalent then that they overshadowed most childhood diseases and genetic disorders. Furthermore, by the mid-nineteenth century only half of the mothers survived beyond their thirty-fifth birthday (many children with Down Syndrome are born to older mothers). In addition there was a high infant mortality and most likely the majority of children with Down Syndrome died during infancy or early childhood.

The first description of a child presumed to have Down Syndrome was given by Esquirol in 1838. Eight years later Seguin described a patient with features suggestive of Down Syndrome and called it "furfuraceous idiocy." In 1866, Duncan noted a girl "with a small round head, Chinese looking eyes, projecting a large tongue who only knew a few words." That same year, John Langdon Down published a paper describing most accurately some of the characteristics of this syndrome which today bears his name. Down mentioned: "The hair is not black as in the real mongol but of a brownish color, straight and scanty. The face is flat and broad. The eyes are obliquely placed. The nose is small. These children have considerable power of imitation."

Although children with this syndrome had been recognized by others prior to his report, Down deserves credit for describing some of the classical features and thus distinguishing these children from others with mental retardation, in particular those with cretinism (children with a congenital thyroid condition). Down's great contribution was his recognition of the physical characteristics and his description of the condition as a distinct and separate entity.

Along with many other contemporary scientists of the mid-nineteenth century, Down was undoubtedly influenced by Charles Darwin's book, *Origin of Species*. In keeping with Darwin's theory of evolution, Down believed that this condition presented a reversion to a primitive racial type. Recognizing a somewhat Oriental appearance in the individuals he observed, Down coined the term "Mongolism" and inappropriately called the condition "Mongolian idiocy." Today we know that the ethnic considerations and racial implications are incorrect. For this very reason, but also because of the negative connotation of the terms Mongol, Mongoloid, and Mongolism, such terminology should be avoided. To call a child with Down Syndrome a Mongoloid idiot is not only a most demeaning insult but also an incorrect description of a child who, although retarded, is first and foremost a child who in most instances is capable of learning and functioning in society.

Subsequent to Down's report there were many clinical studies and publications describing in additional detail the various abnormal findings in Down Syndrome. The question of what causes Down Syndrome was discussed in many medical reports. Advances in technology in the mid 1950s allowed more accurate studies of human chromosomes and it was found that children with Down Syndrome had one small additional chromosome.

Thus, it has only been in the past two decades that scientists have unraveled some of the basic mysteries concerning Down Syndrome. There are still many unknown aspects such as what are the mechanics leading to the additional chromosome or what causes the mental retardation. These questions will require further research for us to arrive at a better understanding of the condition.

5

THE CAUSE
OF DOWN SYNDROME

Siegfried M. Pueschel

When a child with Down Syndrome is born, parents inevitably ask: "How did it happen? What have I done? Why did it happen? Why? Such questions have been asked over and over again by many parents, forcing investigators to search for answers in order to elucidate the cause of Down Syndrome.

Since Down Syndrome was first described more than a century ago, many theories have been postulated about its cause. Astute observations were made by some scientists, but misleading thoughts on the causes of Down Syndrome were also put forward by other workers in the field. Some observant physicians correctly recognized that the mothers of children with Down Syndrome were often at an advanced age at the time of the child's birth. Some thought that the time of bodily maldevelopment of the child must be in the early part of pregnancy, and others felt that certain genetic aspects were probably involved. More often, however, unsupported reports, speculations, and misconceptions led to such untenable hypotheses that alcoholism, syphilis, tuberculosis, or a regression to a primitive human type were all causes of Down Syndrome. Many more hypotheses concerning the causes of Down Syndrome were discussed during the past decades, yet most often they had neither a scientific basis nor did they make any sense considering our present state of knowledge.

By the early 1930s, some investigators suspected that Down Syndrome might be due to a chromosomal problem. However, at that time the technology of examining chromosomes was not advanced enough so that this theory could be proven. When, in 1956, new laboratory techniques were developed that allowed scientists to visualize and better study chromosomes,* it was found that instead of the previously assumed number of forty-eight, there were forty-six chromosomes in each human cell. Three years later, in 1959, Lejeune reported his discovery that the child with Down Syndrome had one extra, small chromosome. He observed forty-seven chromosomes in each cell instead of the normal forty-six chromosomes, and instead of the ordinary two #21 chromosomes he found three #21 chromosomes which led to the term Trisomy 21. Subsequently, geneticists detected that, although an extra, small chromosome was most often present (Trisomy 21), there were also other chromosomal problems that were clinically associated with Down Syndrome, namely, translocation and mosaicism.

Let us try to explain these chromosomal abnormalities in a little more detail.

---

*Chromosomes are tiny rod-like structures which carry the genes; they are inside the nucleus of each cell and can only be identified during a certain phase of cell division by means of microscopic examination.

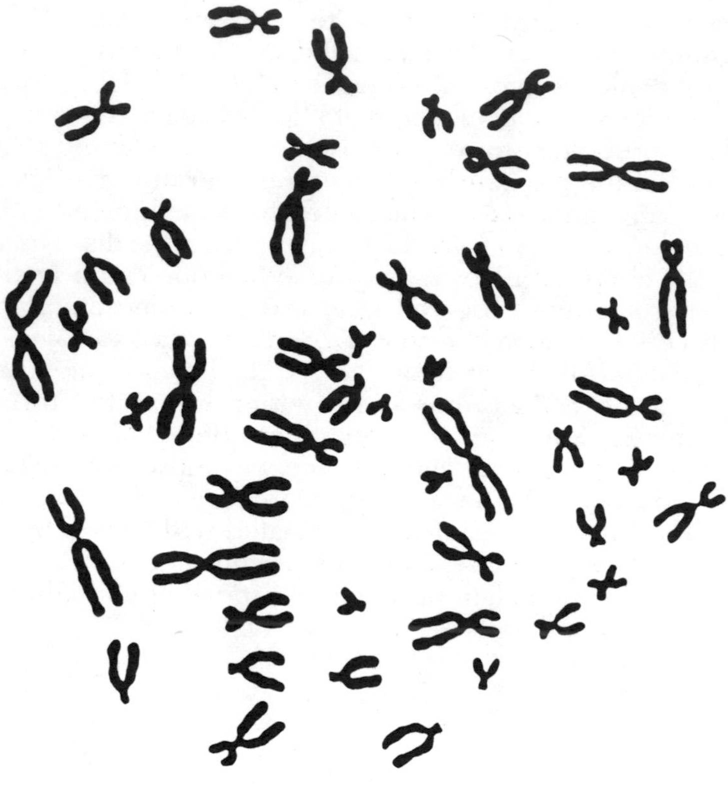

Figure 1
Human chromosomes as seen through the microscope.

There are normally forty-six chromosomes in each cell, as seen in figure 1. These chromosomes can be arranged in pairs as depicted in figures 2 and 3. There are the sex chromosomes which are XX in the female and Xy in the male. The other chromosomes are called autosomes. Half of each individual's chromosomes are derived from a father's germ cells and the other half from a mother's. Germ cells only have half of the number of chromosomes found in an ordinary cell; twenty-three chromosomes are in the egg and twenty-three chromosomes are in the sperm. Under normal circumstances, when sperm and egg are united at the time of conception, there will be a total of forty-six chromosomes in the first cell. Ordinarily, this cell will start to divide and continue to do so as shown in figure 4.

However, if one germ cell (egg or sperm) has an additional chromosome, i.e., a total of twenty-four chromosomes and the other germ cell has twenty-three chromosomes, this will lead at the time of conception to a new cell having forty-seven chromosomes (figure 5). If this extra chromosome is a #21 chromosome the individual, if not miscarried, will be born with Down Syndrome. The original cell with forty-seven chromosomes starts to divide to become two exact copies of itself so that each daughter cell has an identical set of forty-seven chromosomes. The process of cell division continues in this fashion. Later, after delivery, the child's blood cells as well as all other cells of his body will contain forty-seven chromosomes, indicating Trisomy 21.

The question is often asked, "How does the extra chromosome get into the cell?" There are three possibilities of how this can happen: It is feasible that faulty cell division takes place in either (1) the sperm, or (2) the egg, or (3) after fertilization during the first cell division.

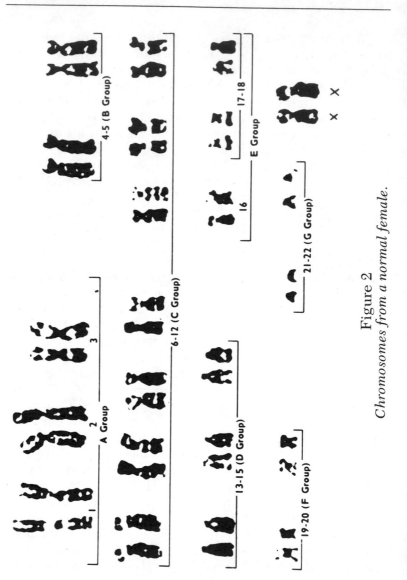

Figure 2
Chromosomes from a normal female.

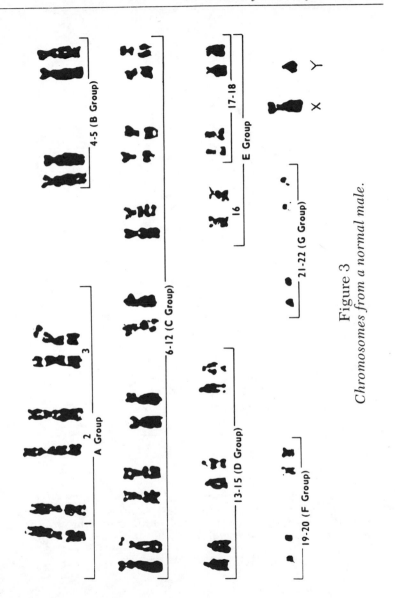

Figure 3
Chromosomes from a normal male.

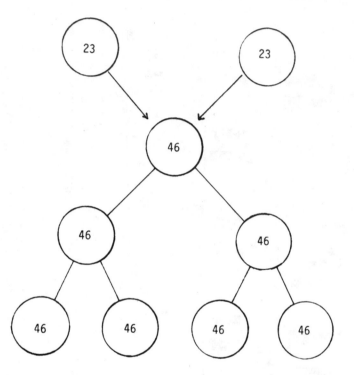

Figure 4
Twenty-three chromosomes derive from each germ cell. At the time of fertilization the first cell has 46 chromosomes. Under "normal" circumstances this cell will continue to divide and in subsequent cell generations each cell will have 46 chromosomes.

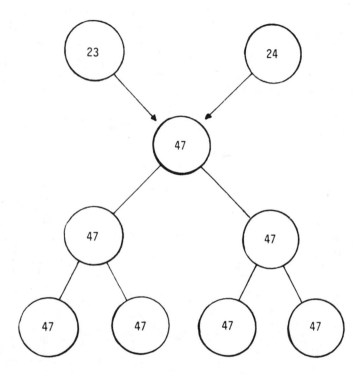

Figure 5
If one of the germ cells (sperm or egg) contributes an extra #21 chromosome then the first cell will have 47 chromosomes and (if not miscarried) a child with Down syndrome will be born.

The mechanism is thought to be the same in all three situations (figure 6). The two #21 chromosomes are somehow "stuck together" and do not separate properly. This process of faulty separation of chromosomes is also known as "nondisjunction" because the two chromosomes do not disjoin or separate as they ordinarily would during normal cell division. Approximately 95 percent of children with Down Syndrome have this form (Trisomy 21) of chromosomal abnormality (see figure 7). Parents should know that once they have a child with Trisomy 21 the chance that any future child may be born with Down Syndrome is 1 to 2 percent.

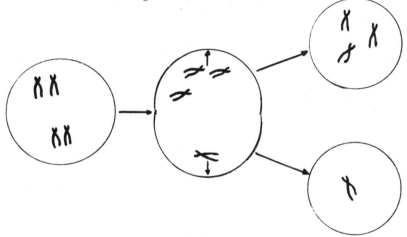

Figure 6

During the process of cell division two #21 chromosomes "stick together" (nondisjunction). In the following cell generation one cell will have one chromosome less (this is not a viable cell) and the other cell will have one additional chromosome.

For demonstration purposes only two pairs of chromosomes are shown here.

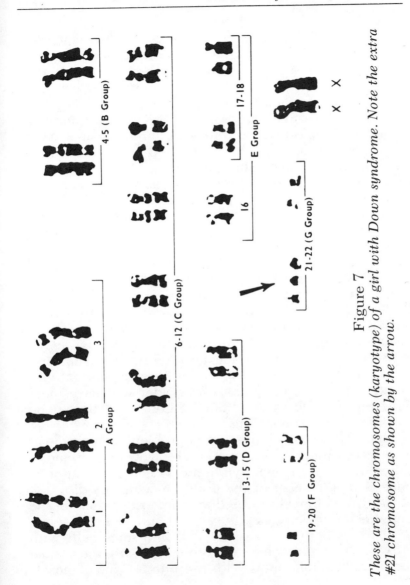

Figure 7

These are the chromosomes (karyotype) of a girl with Down syndrome. Note the extra #21 chromosome as shown by the arrow.

In another 3 to 4 percent of children with Down Syndrome, one finds a somewhat different chromosomal problem. While the total number of chromosomes in the cells of these children is forty-six, the extra #21 chromosome is here attached to another chromosome; but again there are three #21 chromosomes present. The difference in this instance is that the third #21 chromosome is not a "free chromosome," but is attached (translocated) to another chromosome usually from the D or G group. In figure 8 the extra #21 chromosome is translocated to a #14 chromosome. It is important to find out whether or not a child has this so-called translocation type of Down Syndrome, since in approximately one-third of these children one parent is a "carrier." This parent will be perfectly normal physically and have the "normal amount" of genetic material, yet two of his or her chromosomes are attached to each other (as in the baby) so that the total number of chromosomes in this person will be forty-five instead of forty-six. Such a person is called a "balanced carrier" or a "translocation carrier." While the joint chromosomes in the translocation carrier do not alter the normal function of the genes or cause any abnormalities, there is a risk that the carrier will have more children with Down Syndrome. Parents will then need specific genetic counseling.

The third type of chromosomal problem, which is least commonly observed in the child with Down Syndrome, is called mosaicism Down Syndrome, which occurs approximately in 1 percent of the children with this disorder. Mosaicism is thought to be due to an error in one of the initial cell divisions, as you see in figure 9. Later, when the baby is born, one usually will find some cells with forty-seven chromosomes and other cells with the normal number of chromosomes. This presents a "kind of mosaic

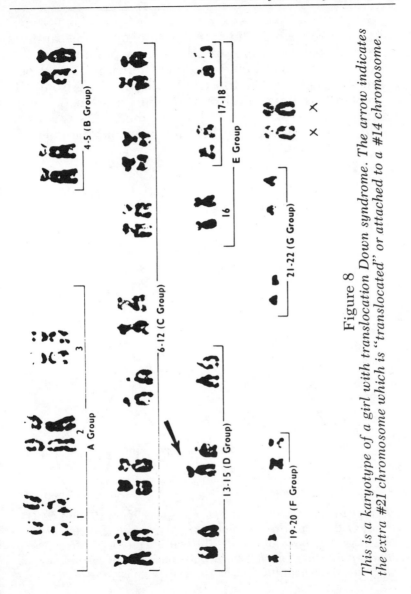

Figure 8

This is a karyotype of a girl with translocation Down syndrome. The arrow indicates the extra #21 chromosome which is "translocated" or attached to a #14 chromosome.

picture"; therefore, the term mosaicism. Some authors reported that these children have less pronounced features of Down Syndrome and that their intellectual performance is better than those of children with Trisomy 21.

Regardless of type (Trisomy 21, translocation, or mosaicism), it is always the #21 chromosome which is responsible for the specific physical features and mental defi-

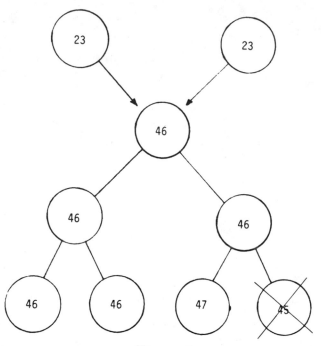

Figure 9

In mosaicism the "accident of nature" (nondisjunction) is thought to occur during one of the early cell divisions. When this infant is born one will find some cells with 46 chromosomes and others with 47 chromosomes. Cells with 45 or less chromosomes usually do not survive.

ciency observed in the majority of children with Down Syndrome. Yet, it is not known in what way this extra chromosome interferes with the development of the unborn child with Down Syndrome, leading to the physical characteristics, or how the deleterious effect on brain function comes about.

Mothers often feel guilty that something they might have done during pregnancy may have caused a baby to have Down Syndrome. Since it is thought that the extra #21 chromosome is present in sperm or egg prior to conception or that an error in early cell division is responsible for the extra #21 chromosome, it cannot be the fault of the mother or the result of anything she did or did not do during pregnancy which led to the child's problem.

In recent years new theories about the causes of Down Syndrome have been proposed, such as radiation and X-ray exposure, administration of certain drugs, and specific viral infections. While it is theoretically possible that those circumstances could lead to chromosomal problems, there is no evidence that any of these situations ever have been directly responsible for the child having Down Syndrome.

Other investigations attempting to explain the faulty cell division which subsequently leads to Down Syndrome have not been helpful in elucidating this problem. At the present time, we just do not know what makes cells divide incorrectly or why chromosomes do not separate properly. It is hoped that future investigations will bring forth new knowledge to shed light on the unknown factors involved.

It is a well-known fact that the occurrence of Down Syndrome is associated with the age of the mother—the older the mother, the greater the risk of having a child with Down Syndrome (see figure 10). Therefore, it is recommended at the present time that mothers over the age of thirty-five undergo a prenatal test (amniocentesis). During this procedure some fluid which surrounds the baby in the mother's womb is obtained with a syringe during the fourteenth to sixteenth week of pregnancy. Should the results of this examination be normal, as one would expect in the majority of situations, such information would be of great value to parents since they could

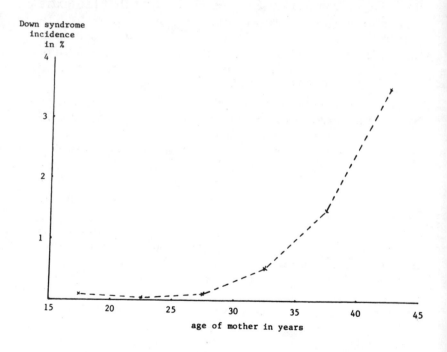

Figure 10

Relationship between maternal age and incidence of Down syndrome. As noted, the older the mother the greater the risk of giving birth to a child with Down syndrome.

then look forward during the remainder of the pregnancy to the birth of a child with normal chromosomes. Should this test show, however, that the baby has Down Syndrome or any other chromosomal anomaly that is likely to cause a significant physical or developmental handicap, the parents might decide to have the pregnancy terminated. It is understood that this is a decision to be made by the parents. Such a procedure should never be dictated by the physician. This procedure (amniocentesis) is also recommended when a parent is a translocation carrier or when a family already has a child with Down Syndrome since there is an increased risk of having another child with this chromosomal problem. Again, specific genetic counseling should be sought out.

6

CHARACTERISTICS OF THE CHILD WITH DOWN SYNDROME

Siegfried M. Pueschel

The appearance and functions of every living being are primarily determined by his genes; likewise the physical characteristics of a child with Down Syndrome are shaped by influences from his own genetic material. Since the child inherits genes from both mother and father, he will to some degree resemble his parents. He may have similar body build, color of hair and eyes; and although smaller, he often follows growth patterns observed within his family. Yet, he does not look exactly like his parents, brothers, or sisters because of his somewhat different "genetic makeup." Due to additional genetic material in the form of an extra chromosome #21, the child with Down Syndrome has a number of bodily characteristics which make him look somewhat different from other children. Since this extra #21 chromosome is found in cells of every child with Down Syndrome, it exerts its body-forming influence similarly in all the children. Therefore, children with Down Syndrome have many physical features in common and look somewhat like each other.

The genes from the additional #21 chromosome are responsible for the altered development of certain body parts during the very early state of the unborn baby's (embryo's) life. We have no insight as to how these changes come about, in what way genes from the extra chromosome interfere with the normal developmental sequences, or how structural changes are induced. We cannot explain why some children with Down Syndrome have certain features or conditions and others who also have the extra chromosome do not. For instance, we do not know why approximately one-third of the children have congenital heart defects and the remaining two-thirds are spared this problem. Much work needs to be done to study these questions, work which hopefully will lead to a better understanding of the mechanisms of how our body is shaped during its early development.

In the following paragraphs, the physical characteristics of the child with Down Syndrome will be described. It should be stressed, however, that these characteristics are most often only minor findings and generally do not interfere with the function of the child. The physical features of the child with Down Syndrome will be more important to the physician for diagnostic purposes.

The *head* is somewhat smaller when compared with normal newborns. The back of the head is slightly flattened in most of the children which gives the head a round appearance. The soft spots (fontanels) are frequently larger and it takes longer for them to close. In the midline where the bones of the skull meet (suture line), there is often an additional soft spot (false fontanel). The hair of the child with Down Syndrome often is sparse, silky, and straight.

The *face* of the child with Down Syndrome appears

somewhat flat due to the underdeveloped nasal bone. Usually, the nasal bridge is somewhat depressed, which makes the *nose* appear small and stubby.

The appearance of the *eyes* somewhat resembles oriental features, which is what led early observers to call these babies "Mongoloids." The eyelids are slightly slanted upward as shown in the picture. A skin fold (epicanthal fold) can be seen in many babies at the inside corners of the eyes. Sometimes the eyes are set far apart. The periphery of the iris often has white speckles (Brushfield spots) due to thinning of the iris tissue. Nearsightedness or farsightedness are more often observed in the child with Down Syndrome than in other children. Cataracts and rapid side to side movements of the eye (nystagmus) are also more common in Down Syndrome.

The *ears* are sometimes small, and the top rim of the ear (helix) is often folded over. The structure of the ear is occasionally slightly altered and the ear is low-set in some children with Down Syndrome. The ear canals are narrow. Middle ear infections and fluid accumulation in the middle ear are common, which occasionally may lead to a mild hearing defect in the child.

The *mouth* of the child with Down Syndrome is often kept open, and the tongue may be slightly protruding. As the child with Down Syndrome gets older, the tongue may become furrowed. The lips are often chapped during wintertime. The inside of the mouth is smaller, and the roof of the mouth (palate) is narrower than the normal child's. The eruption of the teeth is usually delayed. Sometimes one or more teeth are missing, and some teeth may be slightly different in shape. The jaw is also small, which leads to occasional crowding of the permanent teeth later. It is said that dental decay is less often observed in children with Down Syndrome. Yet, regular visits to the dentist and dental hygiene are as important as in any other child. With proper dental care and regular brushing of teeth, one can avoid infections and inflammations of the gums (gingivitis) which often have been observed in persons with Down Syndrome where dental hygiene has been neglected.

The *neck* of the child with Down Syndrome might appear somewhat short. In the infant, loose skin folds are often noted at both sides of the back of the neck which becomes less prominent or may disappear as the child grows.

The *chest* on occasion has a peculiar shape in that the child may have a depressed chest bone (funnel chest), or the chest bone might be sticking out (pigeon chest). In the child who has an enlarged heart due to congenital heart disease, the chest might appear fuller on one side.

In 30 to 40 percent of children with Down Syndrome, *heart* defects are found. A variety of defects have been described, including a hole between the chambers of the heart, abnormalities of vessels or valves, and a combination of various similar problems. Sometimes the heart defect is not readily recognized at the time of birth and might be detected during the first few months of life. Occasionally the heart problem is so severe that children will develop heart failure, which means the heart is too weak to pump enough blood into the vessels of the body. In these instances, specific medications will be given to a child in order to strengthen the heart muscle and to avoid increased fluid in the body.

In approximately 10 to 20 percent of children with congenital heart defects, the defect might be so severe that it is not compatible with life. Those children might not survive beyond the first years of life. Usually a heart specialist will regularly follow children with congenital heart problems. He will inform parents whether the defect is small and will not cause difficulties, whether the child is in need of medications to help the heart to perform more efficiently, or whether heart surgery might be indicated. Significant progress in heart surgery makes it possible for the majority of heart defects to be surgically repaired if this is indicated.

Should your child have a congenital heart defect, you might hear your doctor say that your child has a loud heart murmur. This might be due to blood rushing through a hole between the chambers, to a faulty functioning valve, or to a narrowing of the large vessels. In contrast to such loud murmurs heard in children with congenital heart defects, soft, short, and low-pitched heart murmurs are often heard during the examination of children who have normal hearts. These "mild" or functional murmurs do not signify a heart problem.

The *lungs* of the child with Down Syndrome are usually not abnormal. Some children, in particular those with congenital heart problems, have frequent respiratory infections and sometimes develop pneumonia. With proper medical treatment, these infections can be controlled. Many children with Down Syndrome, however, have no more frequent upper respiratory infections and common colds than other children.

The *abdomen* of children with Down Syndrome ordinarily does not show any abnormalities. Often the abdominal muscles are somewhat weak and the abdomen might be slightly sticking out. The midline of the abdomen is at times protruding because of poor muscle development in this area. More than 90 percent of these children have a small rupture at the navel (umbilical hernia) which usually does not require surgery and does not cause any difficulties later. Most often these hernias close spontaneously as the child grows. The inner organs—such as liver, spleen, and kidneys—are most often normal. In a few children there might be a blockage of the bowels (duodenal stenosis or *atresia*). This can be repaired by a relatively uncomplicated surgical procedure during the newborn period.

The *genitals* of boys and girls are unaffected in the majority of children. They might at times be somewhat small. Occasionally in boys the testicles may not be found in the scrotum during the first few years of life, but may be in the groin area or inside the abdomen.

The arms and legs, *extremities*, are usually of normal shape. The hands and feet tend to be small and stubby. The fingers might be somewhat short, and the fifth finger is often curved slightly inward. In nearly 50 percent of children with Down Syndrome, a single crease across the palm is observed on one or both hands. Fingerprints (dermatoglyphics) are also different from those of other children and have been used in the past to identify children with Down Syndrome. A skin fold between the fingers and toes (webbing or syndactyl) is more often noted in the child with Down Syndrome than in other children. The toes of the child with Down Syndrome are usually short. In the majority of children there is a wide space between the first and second toe with a crease running between them on the sole of the foot. Many children with Down Syndrome have flat feet because of the laxity of muscles and tendons. In some instances an orthopedic specialist might advise that the child wear corrective shoes. In other children there will not be any need for special shoes. Because of the general laxity of tendons and the weak muscles (reduced muscle tone) the child is loose jointed. Ordinarily, this will not cause any problems except when a joint comes out of place (dislocation) as sometimes happens with the kneecap (patella). This requires surgical correction in most instances. Although the hip joints are somewhat differently structured, hip problems are not often encountered in children with Down Syndrome. Many infants with Down Syndrome have poor muscle tone, reduced muscle strength, and limited coordination of the muscles.

The *skin* is usually fair and may have a "mottled" appearance during infancy and early childhood. During the cold season, the skin is often dry, and hands and face may chap more easily than other children's.

While the above-mentioned features are commonly found, there are in addition, other rare congenital problems in children with Down Syndrome and long lists of those "anomalies" have been described in the medical literature. As said before, most of the observed physical findings do not interfere with the development and health of the child. For example, the incurved little finger will not limit the function of the hand, nor will the slanting of the eyelids decrease a child's vision. Other defects, however, such as severe congenital heart defects or the blockage of the bowels, are serious and require prompt medical attention. It is important to know that many of the above described physical features may also be found in other handicapped children and occasionally in normal children.

Not every child with Down Syndrome has all the mentioned characteristics. Certain features may be present in one child and absent in another. Some characteristics which are more prominently developed in a particular child might be less apparent in another. Thus, while children with Down Syndrome can be recognized because of their similar physical appearance, not all such children will look the same. Moreover, some of the features of the child with Down Syndrome will change over a period of time.

7

AN OVERVIEW
OF DEVELOPMENTAL
EXPECTATIONS

Claire D. Canning and Siegfried M. Pueschel

One of the most interesting observations to the parents of a large family is the uniqueness of each child. Brothers and sisters may have strong familial resemblance and may display similar behaviors, but each is a distinct human being different from the other. These very differences can make for a beautiful harmony, an interaction of strengths, weaknesses, joy, and humor that make life such a constant challenge.

The diversity of biological factors, functions, and accomplishments that exist in all human beings is also present in our children with Down Syndrome. In fact, we observe a greater variation in nearly all aspects of their lives. Their physical growth pattern ranges from the very short child with an almost dwarflike appearance to the child with above average height, from the very slim and frail child to the heavy and overweight one. Also, their physical features vary considerably. Some children display only a few of the characteristics, while in other children, many or all of the features may be present. Moreover, the intellectual abilities and the mental development in children with Down Syndrome span a wide range between severe retardation and normal intelligence. We also have learned that their behavior and emotional disposition vary significantly; some children may be placid and inactive, while others are aggressive and hyperactive.

Hence the stereotyped picture portrayed in the past of the short, obese, unattractive individual, with open mouth and protruding tongue, severely retarded and stubborn, is certainly not a true description of the child with Down Syndrome as we know him.

Unfortunately, until recently most articles and reports on Down Syndrome presented data predominantly obtained on institutionalized populations. Based on such information, parents often were given a poor prognosis. One of the authors, Claire Canning, recalls a sad experience after her child was born. She obtained a textbook on "Mongolism," an abysmally discouraging study of unfortunate and almost subhuman people accompanied by even more bleak photographs. She carefully hid this book from her family so that they, too, would not know her anguish. She soon found out that they, in turn, were reading it and hiding it, each perhaps hoping that this "terrible affliction would somehow be made right."

Let us, together, try to dispel misleading reports of the past. Let early intervention, environmental enrichment, and appropriate education, as well as guidance provided to the families, enhance the children's lives.

In the future, parents must obtain more accurate and encouraging information. In fact, the whole purpose of this book is to tell parents that there is hope; that the child with Down Syndrome is, first and foremost, a human being with all humanity's inherent strengths and weaknesses; that we do see a future for our children with Down Syndrome.

Our information here is based on newer studies of children who have been reared in the loving and protected atmosphere of the home. We believe that we can project a truer picture of what one can expect today of children with Down Syndrome.

In the following we will discuss in more detail the observed biological diversity in the child with Down Syndrome and what we may expect regarding his growth, developmental accomplishments, and maturation.

It is generally known that the physical growth is slower in the Down Syndrome child. Our extensive studies support previous reports of reduced growth pattern. From the growth chart (see figure 11) one can, for example, easily identify that the average height of a two-year-old "normal" child is almost 35 inches (89 cm), while the child with Down Syndrome of the same age has an average height of 32 inches (81 cm). As in "normal" children, youngsters with Down Syndrome span a considerable range in height. This variation in growth is determined by genetic, racial, ethnic, and nutritional factors; glandular function, the presence of additional congenital anomalies, and environmental circumstances. It is to be expected that a child with tall parents will be taller than the average child with Down Syndrome. Yet, the undernourished child, the thyroid deficient patient, or the infant with severe heart disease will be expected to be smaller.

At times, parents ask whether there are medications which can accelerate growth. Although several hormones are known to influence growth, we usually do not recommend such treatment. Only if there is a specific indication—for example, stunted growth due to thyroid deficiency—then well-controlled hormone therapy should be forthcoming. We feel that the relative shortness

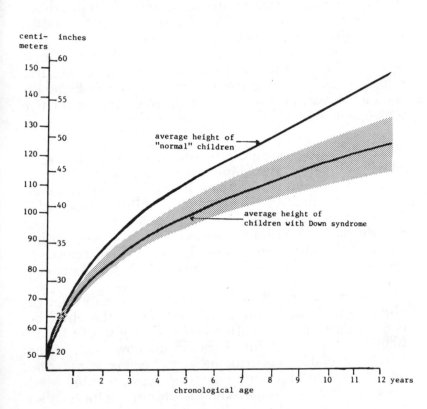

Figure 11

The upper curve shows the average height of "normal" children from birth to 12 years of age. The heavy marked lower curve depicts the average height, and the shaded area the height range of children with Down syndrome.

in children with Down Syndrome is not to their disadvantage. If these children were of average height or taller, then people would expect more of them.

In general, the height of the adult male with Down Syndrome is approximately four feet, ten inches to five feet, four inches while the height of the adult female is somewhat less, between four feet, five inches and five feet, one inch.

Another aspect of growth concerns the weight of the child with Down Syndrome. Since feeding problems are sometimes encountered, there might be reduced weight gain during infancy. In particular, children with additional congenital anomalies, such as heart defects, gain weight slowly. During the second and third years of life, most of the children gradually experience increased weight gain, and from then on overweight may become a problem.

Some parents tend to be overprotective and offer the child an increased amount of food. Once the child becomes accustomed to eating and snacking it will be difficult later to control this "habit." Somehow, one does not look as favorably on carrot sticks and celery as one does on a wedge of chocolate cake or a brownie. One tends unconsciously to compensate the children with goodies, because they cannot run or perform as quickly as other children. Unfortunately, as one does this, the child will move less quickly because extra weight will further lessen his agility. What one wants most is to make the child with Down Syndrome as acceptable as possible to society. It is important to begin early to adhere to a proper diet. Good eating habits, a balanced diet, avoiding high-calorie foods, and regular physical activities can prevent the child from becoming obese.

A weight chart of the young child with Down Syndrome is presented in figure 12. Here, the weight gain of the child with Down Syndrome is compared with the average weight of the "normal" child.

Concerned with developmental accomplishments, parents often ask when their child will be able to sit by himself or when he will finally walk. Answers to these

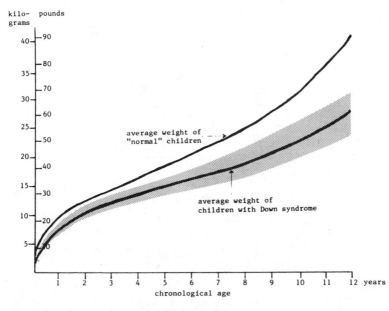

Figure 12

The upper curve represents the average weight of "normal" children from birth to 12 years. The heavy marked lower curve shows the average weight and the adjacent shaded area the weight range of children with Down syndrome.

TABLE I
Developmental Milestones

	DOWN SYNDROME CHILDREN		"NORMAL" CHILDREN	
	average	range	average	range
smiling	2 months	1½ to 4 months	1 month	½ to 3 months
rolling over	8 months	4 to 22 months	5 months	2 to 10 months
sitting alone	10 months	6 to 28 months	7 months	5 to 9 months
crawling	12 months	7 to 21 months	8 months	6 to 11 months
creeping	15 months	9 to 27 months	10 months	7 to 13 months
standing	20 months	11 to 42 months	11 months	8 to 16 months
walking	24 months	12 to 65 months	13 months	8 to 18 months
talking, words	16 months	9 to 31 months	10 months	6 to 14 months
talking, sentences	28 months	18 to 96 months	21 months	14 to 32 months

and other questions relating to the child's motor development are provided in Table 1. The data presented here are derived from our own longitudinal studies as well as from recent reports on motor development in young children with Down Syndrome who are reared in the home. Again, we provide comparable data of "normal" children's development. As mentioned before, there is a wide range in developmental accomplishments. A variety of factors such as congenital heart defects or other interfering biological or environmental problems may be responsible for the marked delay in motor development in some children. In a subsequent chapter, we shall discuss in more detail the motor behavior and approaches to enhancing the motor development of the child with Down Syndrome.

Similar observations were recorded for certain self-help skills and are outlined in Table 2. Of course, the readiness of the child, his maturational level, and the approach to training of such skills are important factors that have to be taken into consideration.

As in many areas of development, the intellectual abilities of the child with Down Syndrome have always been underestimated in the past. Recent reports, as well as our own investigations, negate previous impressions that children with Down Syndrome are usually severely or profoundly retarded. The accompanying figure 13 shows that the majority of children with Down Syndrome function in the mild to moderate range of mental retardation. Some children even have been found to be functioning intellectually in the borderline range and only a few children are severely retarded.

Another misconception refers to the gradual decline of cognitive function of children with Down Syndrome over a period of time. This was not observed in our group of

TABLE II
Self Help Skills

	DOWN SYNDROME CHILDREN		"NORMAL" CHILDREN	
	average	range	average	range
eating				
finger feeding	12 months	8 to 28 months	8 months	6 to 16 months
using spoon/fork	20 months	12 to 40 months	13 months	8 to 20 months
toilet training				
bladder	48 months	20 to 95 months	32 months	18 to 60 months
bowel	42 months	28 to 90 months	29 months	16 to 48 months
dressing				
undressing	40 months	29 to 72 months	32 months	22 to 42 months
putting clothes on	58 months	38 to 98 months	47 months	34 to 58 months

more than a hundred children with Down Syndrome whom we have followed for several years (see figure 14). This new information tells us that the future for the person with Down Syndrome is certainly more optimistic today than ever before.

No reliable data are available on the life expectancy of persons with Down Syndrome. Again, previous reports

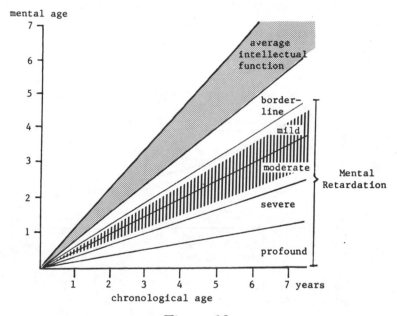

Figure 13

The top shaded area represents children with average intellectual abilities. When children function below "borderline" they are said to be mentally retarded. The majority of children with Down syndrome function in the mild to moderate range of mental retardation as indicated by the vertical bars in this figure.

No reliable data is available on the life expectancy of persons with Down Syndrome. Again, previous reports on this subject are outdated and are no longer valid. There is a dramatic increase in life expectancy since children are treated more effectively for respiratory ailments, heart defects, and other medical problems. Most significant of all is the fact that our children do not grow up in

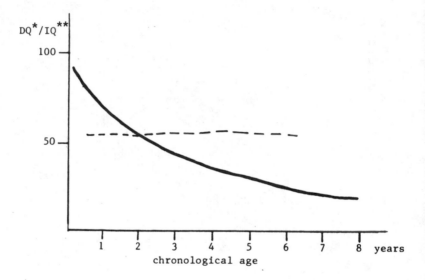

* Developmental Quotient
** Intellectual Quotient

Figure 14

The downward sloping curve represents the decreasing intellectual abilities previously reported by many observers. The interrupted line shows the results of our studies indicating that early intervention, appropriate special education, and home rearing of children with Down syndrome have a positive effect upon their mental function.

institutions, but thrive in an accepting and loving home environment. We assume that life expectancy may be somewhat reduced but not by far as much as was previously reported. Some articles from the literature have referred to the early aging of Down Syndrome individuals, yet, one cannot predict early in life which child will be so affected later on.

While children with Down Syndrome show delay in all areas of biological function, they do make steady progress in their overall development. We know that they possess definite strengths and talents that are an absolute joy to perceive. Their sensitivity, their awareness of the feelings of others, their overall social development, and their sense of humor can bring so much happiness and satisfaction to their families and friends.

While there may be periods of apparent developmental standstill in some children, we usually observe significant developmental advances which both parents and professionals would never have expected in past decades.

Though comparison of various developmental parameters and administering of tests are invaluable to research, there is in each human being something intangible that transcends intelligence quotients and other developmental measures. It is a knowledge that life can be enhanced by optimism, love, and acceptance. Coupled with the support of loving families, hard work of professionals creating innovative programs, and research in biomedical and psychoeducational areas, the future has never been brighter for the child with Down Syndrome.

8

EARLY DEVELOPMENTAL STIMULATION

Elizabeth Zausmer

A child is born with everything needed for contentment, at least during the first stage of life. The newborn sleeps soundly, particularly after a satisfying meal. Sound and visual stimuli enrich his waking hours while being held close, rocked, and fed may supply a multiple of pleasant experiences. Any surplus energy is spent on moving his arms, legs, and trunk. These activities not only please the infant, but bring about increased attention from a parent or other care provider.

But, as so often in life, the rich get richer and the poor get poorer. The normal, healthy child displays a sense of well-being and joy by cooing, kicking, and laughing. His parents, in turn, respond with expressions of love, interest, and provision of a variety of stimulating experiences. The child with a physical or mental handicap frequently cannot evoke the same or even similar reactions in those who surround him. Such an infant may disappoint his parents who in turn may feel deprived. The infant's appearance might not resemble what they dreamed he would look like. In addition, there may be feeding problems. A mother may interpret her child's inability to suck well as a rejection of her, rather than weakness of the muscle he needs to suck or swallow.

Parents and siblings may miss the liveliness and

smoothness of movements which are so typical for the normal infant. The movements of the child with Down Syndrome usually tend to be fewer and slower; they sometimes leave an impression of apathy. But, one has to remember that the child with muscle weakness has to work hard to achieve a result made with little effort by the "normal" child. Sensory stimuli, such as voice, touch, and color also have to be more intense to make an appropriate impact on the infant with Down Syndrome.

The voluminous literature on early intervention and extensive personal experience indicates that physical and mental retardation of the child with Down Syndrome can be modified by competent management and training. Specifically, early intervention can focus on improving an infant's sensory-motor and social development. It may also influence more complex learning processes. In recent years, psychologists and educators have generally agreed that it is the quality rather than the sum total of stimulation that shapes the physical and mental development of the young child. It is, therefore, the structure and the content of a stimulation program that should be emphasized rather than the indiscriminate use of nonspecific stimuli. This is particularly important in planning a stimulation program for the young child with Down Syndrome. Although it is true that this group of children shares many specific developmental handicaps, it is equally true that wide differences are found with regard to their specific capabilities as well as their shortcomings.

The motor development of normal children follows a fairly typical sequence: first comes rolling over, followed by sitting, creeping, standing, and walking. Later we observe more complex activities such as running, climbing stairs, jumping, and skipping. Manipulatory skills also emerge in given sequences such as holding, squeezing, reaching, pulling, and pushing. These skills, together with others in the cognitive and social areas, are gradually combined into activities which allow the child to explore both individual objects and his environment in greater depth and detail. Although the stages of development are fairly fixed, efficient learning, training, and practice of such basic functions contribute to the mastery of physical skills.

If the learning of such activities in the "normal" child requires a good deal of practice and experience, how much more work, patience, and training are needed in the child with Down Syndrome! The latter has to overcome a number of hurdles that slow down the pace of his acquisition of motor skills.

Muscle weakness and poor muscle tone (hypotonia) are in part responsible for the inefficient use of the limbs and trunk, particularly when tasks involve the lifting of body weight against gravity (jumping, hopping, climbing), lifting a load, or working against resistance (pushing an object, pedaling a bicycle).

Increased range of motion in joints (hyperflexibility) is somewhat the cause of instability of joints, particularly the knee and ankle joint. Thus, the child with Down Syndrome may be likened to a person with weak or lax ligaments who does not have the stability to jump well or to hop on one foot.

The curiosity and initiative that are typical of a bright normal youngster are often more difficult to elicit in the child with Down Syndrome due to his slower mental development. This, however, does not mean that the child with Down Syndrome cannot learn.

Learning is a continuous process that starts at birth with the experience of sucking, touching, turning, and lifting the head, followed by looking and listening. Although at first such activities come about reflexively without an intentional basis, they are thought to result in pleasurable sensations which the child repeats successfully. For example, looking at bright lights and objects gradually entices an infant to turn his head and follow moving objects or faces. Later, in search of new and more interesting stimuli, the child explores a variety of voices, colors, textures, and shapes. Thus, the infant soon finds out that active efforts lead to various rewards.

In contrast to the common early experiences of the average child, the infant with Down Syndrome is frequently delayed in engaging actively in motor skills like kicking, wiggling, and rolling over. These activities lead to an effective early exploration of the environment and in turn to continued learning. Parents should actively become engaged in helping their child with Down Syndrome in these early learning experiences. The child who is deprived of, or who has limited capacity to, become involved in such satisfying experiences may become frustrated and either give up efforts to learn or continue to repeat over and over those simple activities which previously resulted in some degree of satisfaction and pleasure. Sometimes the child may revert to self-stimulating patterns of behavior such as rocking or banging his head in order to experience some sensory gratification. The unstimulated child may also show frustration and anger by crying, vomiting, or refusing food. In an extreme situation, the child may give up entirely and retreat into an inner shell permitting little or no effective communications with the outside world. These or similar behavior patterns can be avoided in the child with Down Syndrome. Whatever the level of achievement may be at a given time, there are always some sensory, motor, or cognitive tasks that can provide stimulation, experience, and satisfaction. It takes time and knowledge to choose wisely the components of such a program.

The importance of performing physical skills with efficiency may at first not be obvious, particularly if it involves a child's activities. Perhaps it is easier to understand how physical skills are acquired if we remember how long it took us to perfect such skills as swimming, skiing, bowling, or chopping wood. These are skills that are based on previously acquired patterns of movement which were gradually combined into an organized, complex, sequential series of movements. With an improvement of performance, the learner acquires increasing feelings of pleasure, satisfaction, and success. The greater the ease with which a task is performed, the greater the efficiency. In contrast, an inefficient performance leads to failure and subsequently to frustration; from there it is only one short step to giving up. How much more important it is then for the child with Down Syndrome to experience in early life as many pleasurable and efficient movement patterns as possible! They are essential for his development of more complex skills in the future.

Let us now look at various stages in the development of a child with Down Syndrome and analyze some of the factors involved in providing sensory-motor and other learning experiences to help a child attain higher levels of performance and competence.

Positioning and Carrying

The very young infant with Down Syndrome is apt to lie in a somewhat atypical position; the legs are frequently spread apart and rolled outward with the knees bent. This position, if it becomes habitual, may lead to faulty movement patterns in sitting and walking. One way of keeping the legs closer together is to pin together the bottoms of the garment a child wears during his sleeping periods. Thick layers of diapers should not be worn because they tend to keep the infant's legs apart.

Children with Down Syndrome, who frequently have muscle weakness and who are described as "floppy," are often carried in positions that are not conducive to developing better muscle strength. Parents sometimes carry an older infant as if he were still a newborn baby or they cradle the child excessively, thus restricting active movements of his head, trunk, and limbs.

Infants enjoy being picked up and carried around; they let you know by facial expressions or through body movements that they want to be moved about. A child with Down Syndrome may lack some of the initiative, strength, or means of expression to communicate his wishes to you. Therefore, try to interpret his less obvious signals in regard to positioning, handling, and carrying around.

The position in which a child with Down Syndrome is best carried varies from one individual to the next. It depends on the degree of muscle weakness in different body segments, as well as on the overall developmental level. Generally, it can be said that the young infant with Down Syndrome needs slightly more support of the head and trunk than does the normal child. While the head and trunk most likely have to be cradled at first to prevent sagging and wobbling, it is generally not necessary to restrict movements of the arms and legs by "bundling" these limbs while the infant is lying down, being fed, or carried around.

Besides carrying your child in your arms, you may enjoy the use of a baby carrier strapped to your back (papoose style) whenever your child is ready. You may want to change the infant's position from time to time by turning him around in his little seat since looking out at the world is more exciting than facing the parent's back.

Tactile Stimulation

At a very early age the infant responds most to being touched. Touch is a valuable source of information for the infant. Visual and auditory stimulation should preferably be combined with tactile experiences. Probably the most important early sensory experiences for the infant are being handled, held in the parent's arms, changed, bathed, fed, and carried around. During these natural and spontaneous contacts with the body of a parent or caretaker, the infant obtains a good deal of sensory information. Such experiences may feel good or they may be unpleasant. Pleasant early experiences leave a favorable imprint and may contribute to the child's future physical and emotional well-being.

The following suggestions for tactile stimulation are recommended:

1. Place an infant on surfaces of varying textures, rough as well as smooth blankets, and on different kinds of floor coverings or upholstered furniture. The infant's skin should be exposed to these various tactile stimuli.

2. Cover your infant's body with materials of different textures and weights, also both cool and warm garments. Since the infant's level of activity may change under different conditions, you may want to loosen his garments to allow for freer activity or use more restricting garments to elicit stronger movements against resistance.

3. Touch your child in a variety of ways including stroking his skin, rubbing, tapping, gentle tickling and light squeezing.

4. Let the infant touch you. Place your baby's hands on your face, hair, and clothes and on various parts of his own body. Encourage touching by placing his hands on the bottle or breast during feeding. Let the baby feel different shapes and textures of toys.

5. Move the infant's arms and legs. They can be moved in simultaneous or alternate patterns. Children usually respond more actively when movements are accompanied by singing or playing rhythmic tunes.

6. When bathing an infant in tubs or sinks, do not restrict his movements. Encourage splashing and other body movements while in the water. A pleasant and easy way to bring this about is to take your baby along when you take a bath.

Visual Stimulation

Up to a few years ago, it was generally believed that the newborn or very young infant had a very limited capacity to focus on an object and had even less ability to differentiate between various visual stimuli. This point of view has been proven incorrect. Recent experiments have shown that even newborn infants can differentiate between drawings of faces which present normal human features and those which are distorted or scrambled.

We know now that the infant is ready from the time of birth to look, see, and learn. Therefore your choice of learning experiences is an important one. Infants like best to look at human faces. The distance from which a face is to be viewed has to capture and hold a young infant's interest and attention. Generally, a distance of eight to twelve inches seems to work best. If a sound accompanies the visual presentation, the interest seems to be accentuated.

Although at first the infant will spend most of his time looking at objects while lying on his back, you should make additional visual exploration available to him as early as possible by holding him in an upright position or lying him on his stomach or on his side.

It is also important to provide the infant with visual experiences that are attractive and meaningful. For instance, the feeding bottle might be shown to a child from various directions before sucking starts. A rattle can be looked at before being placed in the child's hand. Also, a parent's face can be moved back and forth before coming close enough to be touched.

At this stage of development the infant can also be expected to explore by mouth all kinds of objects. Exploration by mouth is a very valuable experience which should be encouraged during early infancy. When the arms and hands are brought to his mouth, a movement pattern is practiced which serves as a model for most of the manual activities one engages in throughout life.

Oral exploration also encourages movement of the lips, tongue, and other structures of the mouth which are later used in chewing and swallowing as well as in speech. Therefore, "mouthing," at least in the first few months, should not be discouraged, but seen as a valuable source of information for the child's perception of textures, shapes, temperatures, and tastes.

Prior to the start of manipulating objects more purposefully, a child must be able to fixate visually, organize, and attend to an object. He must be able to see what he wants in order to reach for it or to pick it up. Visually handicapped children are often considerably delayed in developing fine motor skills. They need special auditory and tactile training to make up for their visual deficit.

To evoke your child's attention and interest, attach colorful objects above, as well as on, the sides of his crib. Set the scene for him to turn his head and look in various directions. Commercially available mobiles can be used but improvised ones serve the same purpose. Shiny spoons, colorful clothespins, fluttering multicolor tissue paper, and bells attached to a string can all be made up in various combinations and attached to the bed. Leftover patterned materials cut into interesting shapes and sewn on colorful ribbons are preferable to unicolor materials. So, too, are brightly patterned curtains and sheets.

It is also important to realize that new sensations or impressions provide your child with a better learning instrument than do familiar ones. Thus, it is important to bring new stimuli into your child's life from time to time rather than to rely only on those that have already worked well. Whenever possible, place your child outdoors to provide experiences like looking at leaves, feeling a breeze, or listening to a variety of sounds. Such a visual stimulation program provides some basic skills in looking, focusing, and exploring, following an object through a wider visual range, and differentiation between objects. These preparatory skills are needed for the later stages of active, purposeful grasping and reaching.

Auditory Stimulation

The word "language" is used here to indicate a child's capacity to express pleasure, comfort, hunger, pain, and other sensations (expressive language) and to respond in some way to what is being heard (receptive language).

Infants use facial expressions, grunts, babbles, squeals, cries, and other vocalizations as expressive language. They show their reactions to auditory stimuli through various sounds, facial expressions (smiling, blinking), and body movements such as kicking, squirming, or stiffening of the limbs. They react quite differently to a friendly, soothing voice than to one that is harsh or angry.

Generally, parents communicate spontaneously with their babies by producing sounds such as baba, dada, etc. They also repeat vocalizations they hear from their child. The infant with Down Syndrome, however, might produce sounds less frequently and with less variety of expression. His pitch of voice has fewer highs and lows and the whole expressive repertoire tends to be restricted. It seems to make good sense, therefore, to enrich the auditory environment by introducing a greater variety and intensity of vocal and other sounds.

The human voice attracts and holds the infant's attention better than any other auditory stimulus. One soon notices which particular sounds are preferred. If such sounds evoke pleasure and excitement, the infant will most likely engage in kicking his legs, moving his arms, and wiggling his whole body. If the stimuli are very relaxing and soothing, one frequently observes more quiet movements of the limbs, some smiling, and an increase in focusing.

For the purpose of effective stimulation, a wider variety of sound stimulation should be used:

1. Alternating between low and high pitched voice, whispering, whistling, hissing, and blowing;

2. Use of words with a variety of vowels and consonants that produce expressive movements of the face since infants watch facial movements quite attentively;

3. Frequent smiling, laughing, giggling since the infant reacts quite differently to each of these expressions;

4. Use of sounds and words produced with varying speed, rhythm, and sounds which come from different

directions;
5. Singing with varying modulation of voice.

After a short period of auditory stimulation, there should be a period of observation to see how the infant is reacting. If the response is a positive one, namely that the child seems to enjoy the experience, the same type of stimulation should be repeated a few times. If the child produces a new sound, the parent should imitate it. Wait for a while to give ample opportunity to initiate such communication. You must not forget that your child derives just as much pleasure from hearing you respond to his attempts at making contact as you do when he responds to you.

Frequently for children with Down Syndrome, a combination of strong visual, auditory, and tactile stimulation has to be used to elicit adequate responses. Cuddling, clapping of hands, tapping the skin, gentle tickling or stroking, as well as moving the arms and legs, are some of the ways which have been used to combine tactile stimulation such as talking, singing, playing recorded music, and attaching bells to wrists or ankles.

The most important aspect of any stimulation program is to respond positively to those reactions which show that the infant has engaged in some activity resulting in a new learning experience. Even unimpressive and slow progress may ultimately add up to a point where they may make a difference in the capacity to cope better with the number of tasks which most children with Down Syndrome are able to learn.

9

GROSS MOTOR DEVELOPMENTAL STIMULATION

Elizabeth Zausmer

Head Control

Probably the most important goal in the initial phase of an early intervention program is the attainment of good head control. Before an infant has achieved this stage of development, it is generally very difficult to start working on more advanced developmental sequences. The infant finds it a lot easier to lift his head when lying on his stomach than when lying on his back. Normally, an infant can lift his head while lying on his stomach almost from the time of birth.

Children with Down Syndrome frequently do quite well in this regard. They are apt to lift the head in this position momentarily within the first few weeks of life. The delay in head control becomes more apparent when they are unable to maintain the raised head position for a longer period of time or when they fail to turn the head from side to side. To increase your child's efforts at lifting his head when lying on his stomach, place him face down on a table or bed with the head placed over a well padded edge. In this position, an infant generally makes a maximal effort to raise his head to look at a colorful, attractive toy which is being moved from side to side slightly above him.

When lying on his back, your child also needs extra stimulation to turn the head and to look at objects which are attached to the sides of his bed or strung across the crib. Except for a few smaller things that are fastened to a crib or playpen, the view from the crib should remain open and not be obstructed by padding on all sides, unless this is absolutely indicated for specific reasons. Your child should spend as little waking time as possible in the crib. Being in a playpen, or preferably on the floor, affords a better chance to learn through watching and listening. Once fairly good head control has been achieved, a child is usually ready to start pushing up and rolling over.

Pushing up

At about the time a child holds up his head and looks from side to side while lying on his stomach, the first attempt at pushing up can usually be observed. The child still keeps the elbows bent and leans on his forearms, but soon starts to lift his chest off the surface and arches his back.

Children with Down Syndrome need to strengthen the muscles in their shoulders, backs, and arms. Even at this early stage of development, some variation of the push-up can be introduced to start developing strength in the muscle groups which later will be needed for creeping. Bolsters, blankets, or pillows, shaped into a solid roll, can be placed under the child's hips and stomach; yet the chest should not rest on the bolster. The hips are held firmly with both hands while the child is encouraged to lift his head and upper back. Interesting toys should be placed at an appropriate level in front or slightly above the child's head. They can be moved from side to side to stimulate turning of both head and trunk. Instead of a bolster, a sloping board may be used on which the child lies face down with head and shoulders beyond the edge of the padded board. Excessive arching of the back should be avoided. You may also place your child with his stomach on your lap with shoulders and upper back remaining free of support. Again, encourage lifting of the back and upper part of the trunk. Most likely, the child who pushes up on his arms with the elbows straight is ready to roll over. Some children roll over before they push up.

Rolling over

The motor developmental phase of rolling over is an important one for a child because it expresses the wish and ability to move from one place to another. The child with Down Syndrome may enter this developmental phase at a later age than the average child, and may also remain at this level of activity for a considerably longer period before moving on to the later stages of crawling or creeping.

Parents should recognize that rolling over is a valuable experience and a good preparation for future, more mature motor achievements. You should stimulate rolling over, if it does not occur spontaneously. Place your child on a mat, small rug, blanket, or folded sheet. Two persons, holding the mat at either end, roll the child gently back and forth by tilting the mat from one side to the other. Most infants enjoy this activity; it is a good steppingstone for a more active, voluntary form of rolling. It provides the experience of shifting the weight from one side to the other. It also helps to overcome the child's fear of sudden movements and changes in position.

When the child has become adjusted to being rolled, encourage more active rolling from back to side. A favorite toy is placed at a short distance stimulating a child to turn his head toward the toy to look at it. The child will often reach across his body in order to touch the toy and subsequently start rolling over. You may need to help a little by moving the top leg across the other leg to initiate the movement. If your child enjoys being helped to roll over, a more spontaneous, active movement will follow.

Rolling from stomach to back is a more complicated process because more head control is needed as well as the ability to initiate the movement by pushing up on one arm. However, once your child has started to lift his head and back while lying face down, it usually does not take too long before active rolling in both directions is accomplished.

Rolling over should be encouraged. It is a good exercise for training body control and balance. It is also an early developmental activity which is brought about through a child's initiative, curiosity, and motivation to learn more about his environment.

Sitting

When a very young infant is pulled up to the sitting position his head often wobbles and drops backward. This is called head lag. The child with Down Syndrome maintains a head lag position considerably longer than the "normal" child. This is partly due to weakness of the neck muscles, but it also is due to his general developmental delay. Head lag decreases with maturation, but it is important to encourage good head control in sitting as early as possible. Therefore, one should not let the child's back always rest against the mother's body or against the back of a chair while in the sitting position. Only minimal support should be given to prevent toppling over or sitting with poor posture.

If a child is held firmly around the hips, he will frequently straighten his back to maintain good balance. It may be necessary to put one's hand around the ribs of a child who still has poor balance in sitting. Such firm support frequently controls the wobbling of the head. Gradually, a child will learn to control the muscles of the neck and upper part of the back. The child will then sit with little or no support.

Even the very young infant enjoys being pulled up to a sitting position. When a finger is placed in his palm, his response is one of bending his arms. At a later stage he will attempt to initiate the movement of coming up to sitting. Encouraging a young child to grasp your finger, to bend his elbows, and to pull himself up to sitting develops the muscles of his arms, shoulders, and trunk while it helps to improve head control. However, if there is considerable head lag, the head must be slightly supported to prevent it from dropping backward.

Most infants first sit in bed or on the floor while propping themselves up on their arms, which are placed at their sides or in front of them. Due to muscle weakness, this position is a difficult one to maintain for most children with Down Syndrome. The arms may not be strong enough to carry the weight of the trunk; the back may be rounded and the head may drop forward. Also, in order to maintain balance, the legs usually are spread wide apart.

Postures and positions that are detrimental to the development of motor behavior should be avoided. Rather than permitting a child to sit for long periods of time on the floor, you should choose a sitting position where the hips and knees are bent and held fairly close together, and the trunk is held erect. An infant seat, small chair, or any similar seating arrangement can be improvised in many ways. Sitting on a little chair leads to good postural pat-

The hair often is sparse, silky, and straight.

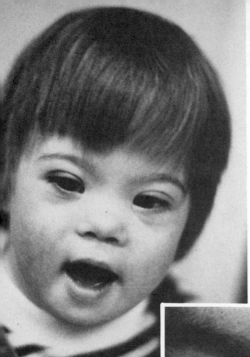

Usually the nasal bridge is somewhat depressed, which makes the nose appear small and stubby.

The periphery of the iris often has white speckles (Brushfield spots) due to thinning of the iris tissues.

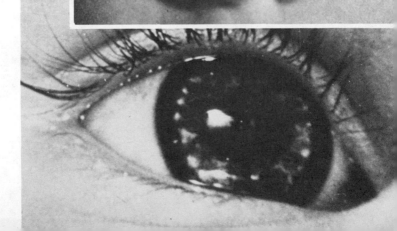

The ears are sometimes small, and the top rim (helix) is often folded over.

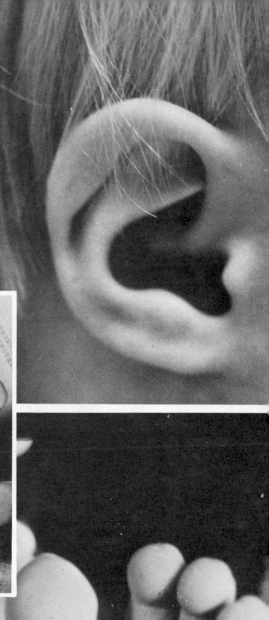

A single crease across the palm is observed in nearly half of the children with Down syndrome.

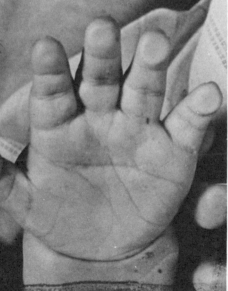

There is a wide space between the first and second toe with a crease running between them on the sole of the foot.

Characteristic resting position of the young infant with Down Syndrome (see page 81)

Placed over a firm pillow, push-ups are started (see page 89)

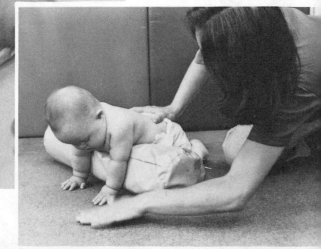

With the trunk off the wedge, a more advanced version of push-off is used (see p. 90)

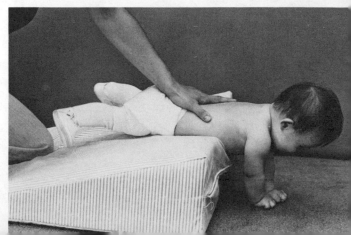

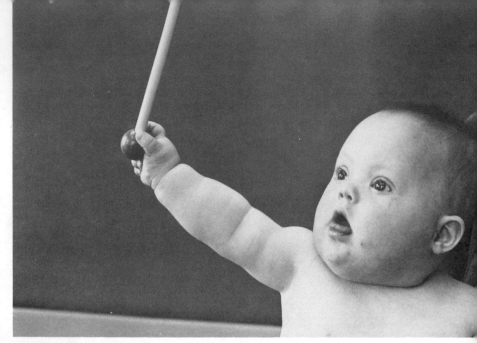

When the child shows readiness for reaching, a toy should be placed in a position which necessitates some effort on his part to obtain it (p. 107)

Sitting: if the child is held firmly around the hips, he will frequently straighten his back to maintain good balance (see p. 92)

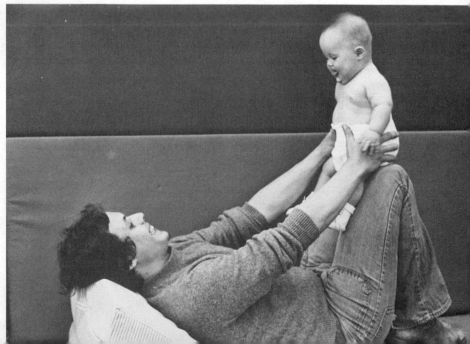

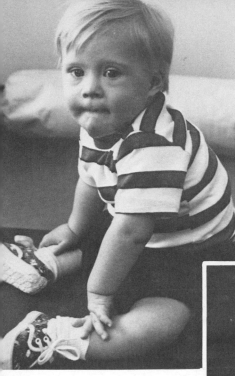

Poor sitting posture, as shown here, should be avoided (see p. 92)

A strap — attached to the chair in seatbelt fashion — stabilizes the hips for good support (see p. 93)

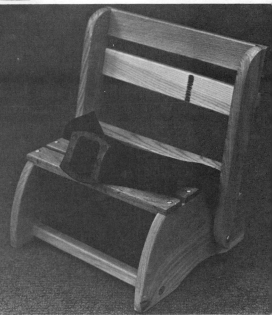

A chair of proper height allows the child to sit straight with legs in good position (see p. 93)

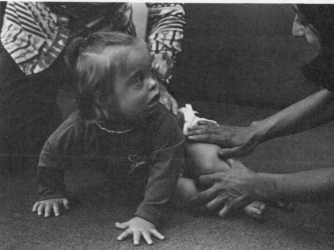

The child is exposed to various changes in body position to encourage adequate balance reactions (see p. 94)

The child will need help in practicing a more normal sequence of movements when learning to sit up (see p. 94)

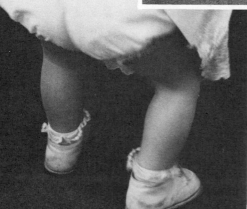

At first, the child is apt to stand with legs too far apart and turned out — but posture can be improved by training (p. 99)

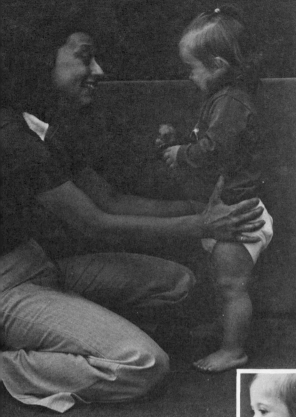

Getting used to stand correctly (see p. 99)

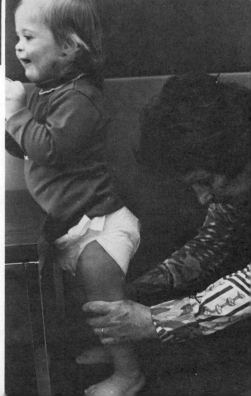

By pushing down gently on the hips, a reaction of resistance is elicited which may result in an improvement of posture in standing (see p. 99)

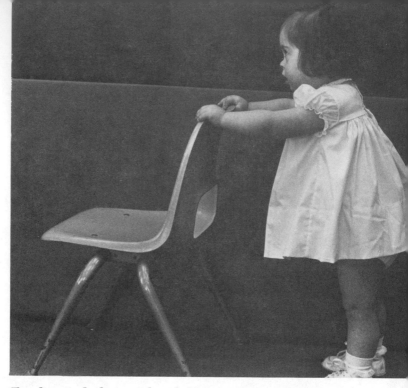

For better balance, the child first pushes a chair (p. 101) . . .

. . . and then takes off on his own (see p. 101) (see p. 101)

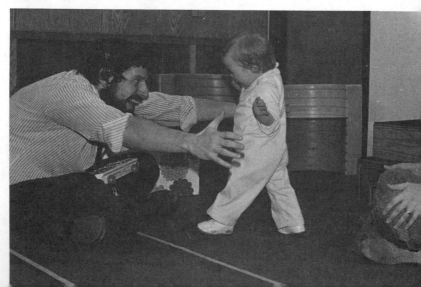

terns of head and trunk control. A chair must always be adjusted to the child's height and body proportions. A child's legs should not be spread apart too widely, and his feet should be placed in a good position on the floor. Such a sitting position gradually enables the child to shift some weight onto his legs and feet, a valuable preparation for future weight bearing in standing and walking.

If your child does not seem to be ready for unsupported sitting, you may attach a strap or belt to the chair for stabilizing his hips. Such a strap should be attached to the chair like the seatbelt in a car, but be sure to avoid placing the strap around the child's stomach or chest. A child who is tied to the back of a chair is apt either to slip down under the strap or slouch forward over it. A bouncer chair has to be elevated appropriately for each individual child. It might help to improve strength in some muscle groups if your child is able to sit with good posture and if his legs are used to push up. However, sitting passively slumped over in a bouncer serves no useful purpose.

With advancing age and maturation, more complex and demanding changes in sitting positions have to be added in order to develop good balance. Balance reactions occur when the body is tilted forward, sideward, or backward, especially when such positions are changed fairly quickly. The following are activities which can be used to elicit balance reactions:

1. Lift and then lower your child while holding him either in the upright or horizontal positions, supporting the infant with your hands around his hips. If this does not seem to be a safe enough hold, place your hands around the child's chest.

2. Lie on the floor with your knees bent. Place your child against or on top of your knees and give support as needed. Rock your child forward, backward, and from

side to side. Move your own knees off and onto the floor (this is also an excellent exercise for your own stomach muscles!).

3. While your child sits on your lap, tilt him gently forward, backward, and from side to side. Prevent excessive wobbling of the head, but don't overprotect by giving too much support to head and trunk. Remember that an improvement in balance can only be brought about if the child makes a strong, active attempt at balancing himself.

Gradually, the above outlined activities, or any others that serve the same purpose, can be increased in complexity, intensity, or duration in order to challenge your child to respond with his full capacity.

From Lying to Sitting

Most children need little practice in learning how to move from the lying to the sitting position. They simply turn on their side, push up on the arms, and there they sit.

In contrast, children with Down Syndrome frequently follow a different sequence of movements. They roll over onto their stomach, then spread their legs so far apart that they hardly need to push up on their arms to raise their trunk off the floor. Although at first, this may be the only possible way for your child to come to sitting without your help, you should discourage such motor development. You and your child should try to practice a more normal sequence. This is done in the following way: the child rolls to the side-lying position. You bend his hips and knees toward his chest. Next, place the child's hand on the floor near the knees. Now help your child to push up and to shift his trunk over the buttock, thus coming to the upright position. Gradually decrease your assistance.

A very important milestone has now been reached, not only in gross motor development, but also in other respects. The youngster can observe what is going on around him. He can reach for objects that were not accessible before; he can lie down and sit up, responding to different situations, and he can roll to a different place and then explore it while sitting. Gravity has for the first time been conquered; your child will be enchanted with this accomplishment—and so will you!

The ability to sit up has opened new horizons for your child. The next stage of gross motor development—not easy to achieve—will be that of crawling and creeping.

Crawling and Creeping

The term "crawling" is used to describe the child who is moving about with his stomach touching the floor. "Creeping" means that the child moves on his hands and knees.

Almost all children crawl before they creep. The child with Down Syndrome may lack sufficient muscle strength in his arms, shoulders, and trunk to come to the hand-knee position, or to maintain such a position for any length of time. Therefore, the stage of crawling may be considerably prolonged. For many children it is easier to crawl backward or to pivot, than to crawl forward.

Sometimes, the lack of motivation to crawl or to creep may retard a child's progress. It is not enough to place a toy on the floor and to assume that your child will be sufficiently interested to go after it. The child with Down Syndrome may not exhibit the same degree of attention, initiative, curiosity, and stamina we find in the nonhandicapped child. Therefore, one must find the maximal and optimal stimuli that work best at a given time and under given circumstances. Once this has been determined, such stimuli should be used until they can be replaced by new stimuli and novel experiences.

Most observations have shown that the color of a toy or other object influences the child's desire to handle it. Although children vary somewhat in their color preference, most prefer orange, red, and yellow to other colors. Whatever the color, an object that moves is most attractive to the young child. Almost all children show heightened attention or excitement when they look at an object that is pulled, swung, moved up and down, twirled, or spun around. Thus, mobiles, toys that bounce on springs, rings or bells attached to strings, and wind-up toys attract the child's attention most.

The child who is well motivated to crawl or creep but lacks sufficient muscle strength to do so may be helped by partially taking his weight off his limbs. Wrap a wide strap or a folded towel around his abdomen, then lift the abdomen slightly off the floor. Initiate the child's creeping movements by tapping lightly on the soles of his feet or by assisting the movements of his arms and legs. Gradually, your child will participate more actively with less support.

A piece of equipment that has been commercially introduced is called a crawligator. It is a plastic board on wheels. The child lies with his stomach and chest on the crawligator. This frees his arms and legs from having to bear much weight. In some selected instances, this temporarily may be a helpful device to encourage your child to start creeping. However, it presents a less voluntary, less active, and less controlled way than the procedure outlined above. If the crawligator or a similar device is used at all, it should be used in relation to the individual child's developmental level, capacity, and needs. Check with a physical therapist before you purchase this piece of equipment.

Creeping upstairs is an excellent way to gain a sense of

balance and to develop good movement patterns. Strangely, a child who does not seem to want to creep on a flat surface will often enjoy creeping up stairs with some help if a toy is placed where it can be seen and eventually reached.

Although some children may not like to creep very much, you may find that if you yourself get into the all-four position on the floor, your child will enjoy moving along with you. If you add a hide-and-seek game, it won't be long before your little one will come creeping around the corner looking for you.

At a more advanced stage of creeping, the action can be enlivened by setting the scene for creeping under tables, beneath chairs, and over boxes which have been turned upside down to create tunnels. To see a child creep heavily all over the house is a wonderful sight. The child has become your companion following you around, eager to see and to be seen.

Kneeling and Knee-Standing

After a child has mastered creeping, he is probably ready to pull up to standing. Most children come to the kneeling position and then use a chair or the leg of a parent to pull themselves up to the erect position. The child with weak muscles may find it difficult to go through such a motor sequence since its successful completion is dependent on muscle strength in his legs, arms, and trunk. It is exactly for that reason, namely to strengthen muscles and to learn to maintain the trunk in the erect position, that training in kneeling is important.

A parent can help a child to come up to kneeling and to maintain this position without fear or discomfort by holding his hips firmly and stabilizing his legs. A toy is placed on a chair or couch to motivate the child to get and stay in this position.

While kneeling, the child's shoulders, hips, and knees should be well aligned. The child who can kneel in this correct weight bearing position has a better chance to develop a good gait pattern. Coming up from kneeling to standing should now be practiced in the manner in which any child would use spontaneously—one leg placed in front. Generally, the preferred leg is used to push up while balance is maintained by holding on to a steady object.

Kneeling is the first weight bearing position to be attained while the trunk is held erect. It is a good preparation for standing and walking because it lowers the center of gravity and thus affords more stability for balance. In kneeling, the child can practice and becomes accustomed to shifting his weight from one leg to the other, the basis of walking.

Standing

Standing is a term which would seem to need no further description. However, in using the word to describe an atypical child's motor behavior, it needs some discussion.

Most children who have learned to pull themselves up proceed rather quickly to stand unsupported for longer periods of time. They rarely spend much time standing before they take off and start walking. Their balance is well established when they have reached this maturational stage, and they progress fairly quickly to unsupported walking. This is why many parents cannot remember at what age their child started to stand, while they are apt to recall without difficulty how old their child was when he took his first step.

Children with Down Syndrome may follow a somewhat different progression of motor development. They stand considerably later than the "normal" child. Usually, they need support for a longer time period before they can stand by themselves. There are many reasons for this delay. Muscle weakness in the antigravity muscles of the legs and the trunk delay the attainment of the erect position. Also, children who have weak muscles are frequently more fearful of standing unsupported. A lack of initiative in trying a new activity may also contribute to the delay.

A child with Down Syndrome will most likely stand at first with his legs spread widely apart and his feet turned slightly outward. This position is almost always spontaneously assumed because it affords better balance and stability. It is a position, however, which should be changed to improve the motor pattern lest the child become used to this rather ungainly and ineffective way of standing.

One of the first steps in encouraging proper standing is to make sure that a child's body weight is carried or shifted onto his legs. The child must acquire the sensation of actually standing on his feet, rather than using his arms to support the weight of his body by hanging on to a support such as a table or chair. One way to achieve proper weight bearing is to push down gently on the child's hips in order to elicit a reaction of resisting, which in turn will straighten his knees and trunk.

One can also convey the sensation of weight bearing by steadying his knees while simultaneously holding his feet firmly against the floor. At first, these exercises can be done while your child leans against a wall or stands in a corner. Gradually, the child will develop confidence in his ability to stand on his own as your support is gradually decreased. To overcome the fear of losing his balance, you might encourage your child to hold a large ball or toy, to beat a small drum, to reach for a suspended toy, to touch your face or hair, or to engage in movements which shift his attention from his legs to a more enjoyable activity. Thus, the child's confidence in standing is slowly developed.

Walking

Although standing and walking are often considered to be one entity, they are quite different phases of motor development. While assuming an erect body position and maintenance of balance are equally needed for both activities, nevertheless a third component is introduced in walking, the ability to propel the body forward.

A child who spontaneously starts to walk has most likely acquired sufficient balance to stand on one leg while the other is swinging forward. The weight can then be shifted to what becomes the supporting leg. This is the reason that during the preceding training for correct standing, a great deal of time was spent on learning to shift the weight from one leg to the other.

For a child with Down Syndrome, walking may present a considerable hurdle. Even after having mastered to stand on both legs without support, standing on one leg appears to be a great deal more difficult. Therefore, the transition from supported to unsupported walking is frequently considerably delayed.

The same postural characteristics of a child with Down Syndrome that were seen in standing may still be present in walking. The legs are spread apart, the knees pointed outward and pushed backward, and the feet are flat on the floor. The previously described measures to avoid or to minimize such faulty postural patterns might again have to be taken.

While almost any child cruises along the wall or around a low table for a short period of time, the child with Down Syndrome often does not dare to take such sideward or forward steps for a long time. A great deal more encouragement, motivation, and support is needed to overcome the fear and apprehension of falling. Although at first the child likes to hang on to a parent's hand, prolonged leading by hand is not the best way to accelerate unsupported walking. If a child is virtually suspended by being led around with his arms held up, his chance of shifting and maintaining the weight on the legs is considerably reduced.

A more appropriate way is to hold your child by the hips or around the waist in order to leave his arms free to swing, carry a toy, or push a chair. Gradually, such support can be reduced and the child will be able to take a few steps from one parent to the other.

Studies published in the last few years have documented that the age at which children with Down Syndrome start walking varies a great deal. It has been claimed that there is a relationship between intelligence and the starting age of walking. However, the onset of walking does not necessarily reflect a child's current level of intelligence, nor does it predict intelligence at a later age. Complicating factors such as cardiac disease and other medical conditions, as well as frequent hospitalizations, are apt to delay developmental milestones. As with "normal" children, one has to be careful not to use the age of walking as an indication of how well the child with Down Syndrome will do at later developmental stages. It should also be understood that gross motor development (sitting, standing, walking) is frequently less delayed than is the acquisition of speech and language.

A careful, early assessment of the characteristics of gait is a most important feature of the child's motor developmental program. The evaluation is usually done by a physical therapist who plans the intervention program best fitted to the special needs of an individual child. Faulty motor patterns should be prevented before they become part of a child's repertoire that may be difficult to correct later on.

Running

In running, the weight is shifted faster from one leg to the other than it is in walking. There is also a need to propel the body forward and to maintain balance during movements performed at greater speed. A certain degree of strength in the calf muscles is needed for the forward thrust of the body. Normally, the swinging of the arms makes running a smooth, rhythmic performance.

The child with muscle weakness frequently encounters some difficulties, both in maintaining the erect position and in propelling the body forward. He may run slowly and awkwardly, barely lifting his feet off the floor while his arms are frequently held at shoulder level for better balance.

The following are a few of the activities which have been successfully used to prevent faulty motor patterns:

1. High stepping or stepping over hurdles such as boxes, boards, rope; lifting knees to chest while running in place; stepping up on high steps, stools, or low chairs.

2. Walking on tiptoes; reaching for toys which are placed at a high level.

3. Balancing on one leg, first with support then gradually with less support; walking on a board placed on the

floor or slightly raised off the floor.

4. Swinging arms in alternate, rhythmic movements; hitting a soft object such as a suspended ball, with alternate arms; throwing a ball with alternate hands; beating a drum with two sticks; marching while tapping one lifted knee with the opposite hand.

For the child who does not move fast or try to start running, one must search for a way to encourage initiative and a sense of competition. Whenever possible, enjoyable group activities should be used. They often result in success. Squatting down and coming up from squatting are activities which strengthen the antigravity muscles of the trunk and legs. Most children enjoy picking up objects from the floor or playing in the squatting position. The child with Down Syndrome frequently prefers to sit down rather than squat, since the latter is a more demanding position to maintain with insufficient muscle strength. Thus, whenever possible, squatting should be encouraged, as well as frequent changes from the sitting to the standing position.

Climbing stairs is another activity which develops balance and strengthens the muscles of the legs. A child with delayed motor development and weak musculature tends to hitch up and down stairs on his buttocks rather than walk erect. Climbing stairs should be practiced early and frequently, first with two-hand support which is gradually decreased to one-hand support, until sufficient balance is present to manage stairs unsupported. At all times, the child should be protected from falling down stairs.

Jumping and hopping are activities which demand a higher degree of balance and propulsion than needed in running. Both are excellent motor activities for a child who needs to develop balance and muscle strength. First, jumping up and down in place may be practiced on an old mattress or a couch. As the child's skill improves, a soft rug should be used. Jumping alone is not much fun, but jumping with parents, siblings, or friends, accompanied by a lovely rhythm, is. Jumping and hopping can also be incorporated into all kinds of games: imitating the movements of animals, jumping along lines drawn on the floor, jumping over obstacles, or jumping down from steps. These are only a few of the many motor skills which prepare a child to handle unexpected changes in body position and speed of movement.

The child who is not very interested in gross motor activities or who finds it physically difficult to engage in more advanced and complex gross motor skills may lack the initiative to try to perform. In the case of a child with Down Syndrome, much more time and practice is needed to bring about a change in interest and attitude. Stronger and more specific directions are used for instruction and correction as well as frequent repetition of smaller segments of a motor activity. Activities should be structured so that they result in success and satisfaction. Failure produces an increasing sense of frustration, and the child soon gives up on striving to perform better. In contrast, the satisfaction in having succeeded and of having pleased a parent or teacher is a very desirable kind of reinforcement. Your child's reward can be a hug, the opportunity to enjoy a special TV program, your taking him to a favorite place, or a chance to play with a favorite toy. Food as a reinforcement should be used as sparingly as possible. Food as the main or only source of enjoyment can all too easily become a set pattern of gratification and satisfaction in later life, resulting in increased weight gain.

Although children with Down Syndrome may not be expected to become great athletes, there is no reason to assume that they cannot achieve a considerable degree of progress in sport or other recreational pursuits. As a matter of fact, their body skills may later be their most valuable means of competition at a time when their intellectual limitations are apt to adversely affect their social contacts and experiences. Even apart from competition, bowling, dancing, swimming, skiing, and other similar activities can enrich a person's life. First and foremost, however, the joy and satisfaction that arises from using one's body effectively will contribute to making a child's future life a more meaningful and rewarding one.

10

FINE MOTOR DEVELOPMENTAL STIMULATION

Elizabeth Zausmer

The hand has frequently been called the instrument of intelligence. Children who are highly skilled in performing complex, fine motor activities are generally found to be intelligent, but those with lesser intellectual capacity can also be trained to become quite efficient in carrying out manual tasks.

During the evolution of man, the ability to use the hand has been linked with the assumption that this would require erect posture, thus freeing the forelimbs for non-weight bearing motor skills. Similarly, an infant first acquires basic and slightly more advanced motor skills such as sitting, creeping, standing and walking, before becoming maturationally ready to engage in fine motor skills of any magnitude or complexity. Such sequential development does not necessarily apply to the child with Down Syndrome who may be held back in gross motor development because of significant muscle weakness, heart disease, or other physical defects. Such a child may be ready maturationally for more advanced, fine motor activities and play before becoming competent in gross motor skills.

A thorough evaluation of the child's vision, attention span, and level of cognitive development is needed.

106

Muscle strength and muscle control of a child's head and arms has to be checked before a home program, geared to the needs of the individual child, can be planned. Whatever the level of your child's ability, fine motor stimulation should combine a variety of learning experiences.

Again, a carefully structured learning situation should be set up for infants at a very early age. At birth and during the first few weeks thereafter, the infant grasps an object that is placed in his hands. This is called "the reflexive grasp." Release does not occur voluntarily; the object is dropped when the fingers relax.

Infants seem to prefer long and slender objects to short, round ones. Handles of spoons, clothespins, rods, and similar objects attract their attention most. When a child shows readiness for reaching, a toy or an object should be placed in a position which necessitates a certain amount of effort on his part to obtain it. On the other hand, the child eventually must be able to get hold of the toy rather than have to give up in frustration. An observant parent will appreciate his child's efforts and offer rewards.

The child who has muscle weakness and needs more stability to carry out motor activities has to be positioned more carefully to make maximum use of all available muscle strength in the arms, shoulder girdle, and trunk. You may want to refer to the previously outlined positions of lying on the side, on the stomach, or sitting, to decide which one is best suited for a specific task. In addition, one can help a child by positioning toys in a way that allows his arms to be supported comfortably so they can be brought in front of him. Such a position also provides a good angle of vision. Sometimes a child is left with toys placed too high on a table, making it difficult for him to reach. If toys are placed too low, poor postural and visual patterns result: sitting with the back very rounded, the head held too close to the play material, or the arms held in cramped positions and unable to move freely.

Young infants initially use raking movements to pick up an object. They take hold of it with the entire hand (palmer grasp). Subsequently, a thumb-index-finger-grasp develops, making it possible to pick up and handle smaller objects. Children with Down Syndrome start later than the average child in swinging the thumb around the palm of the hand. The thumb-index-finger-grasp (pincer grasp) can be practiced by placing and holding your child's thumb and index finger around an appropriate object such as a small block, a paper ball, a bead, or a coin. Gradually, your child will be encouraged to pick up such objects without help. A child who still prefers to use the palmer grasp will start to use the pincer grasp if an object is held out or handed to him rather than placed on a table to be picked up. As your child's dexterity improves, his desire to pick up small objects such as pieces of crackers, cookies, cereal, or raisins can be used to encourage more frequent use of the pincer grasp.

Children with Down Syndrome need extra stimulation, encouragement, guidance, and training in manipulatory skills. They have to be shown how to explore objects with their hands, how to roll a little paper ball in the palm of the hand, and even how to hold on to something that could easily slip out of their hands. Therefore, encourage use of the hands as early as possible.

At the table, let your child with Down Syndrome use his hands to explore different types of food to learn the difference between solids and liquids, warmer and colder foods. Assist him in sticking his finger into applesauce, warm cereal, cold ice cream, sticky marmalade, and peanut butter. Of course, let your child lick all these goodies off his fingers. Once the path from finger to mouth has been well established, finger feeding is soon apt to follow.

Learning to use both hands simultaneously and to transfer an object from one hand to the other occurs quite spontaneously in the "normal" child. However, it needs to be practiced with the child who shows a developmental delay in fine motor skills. Pat-a-cake is a fun way to interest a child in using both hands simultaneously. Hold your child's hand in your own and clap them together while singing or listening to a tune. If the child starts to participate, reward him by smiling and hugging. Decrease your assistance gradually.

Place a large ball between your child's hands. Put your own hands on top of his to convey the feeling of holding firmly and with pressure. Then show how the alternate release and firm grasp differ. Augment this experience by consistently using directions like "hold" and "let go." Put your child's hands on a stick or rod. Show him how one hand alternately releases the hold while the other one maintains the hold. This "trick" seems to speed up the emergence of the skill of transferring an object from one hand to the other.

The use of fingers as separate units (rather than moving all fingers simultaneously) should also be encouraged. The index finger may be used for poking, sticking into a hole, hitting the key of a piano, or pushing a button. Guide your child's hand holding a peg, a ring, or a coin between three fingers. Provide experience in crumpling paper or throwing a block. These are only a few of the activities which should be practiced in order to avoid unnecessary delay in the acquisition of more advanced fine motor skills. During play, finger and hand movements should be carefully observed. Guide your child through the correct movement patterns. This will give him a good model for more independent manipulation in the future.

Normally, an infant learns fairly quickly that an object which is first held in the hand can also be dropped. Children who develop more slowly seem to want to hold on to objects for more extended periods of time. They do not want to give them up. Therefore, they have to be motivated and shown how to open their fingers to let a block or little ball drop. When a toy is dropped into a metal container, rather than into a carton or plastic box, the child can hear the resulting sound. You should also reward him and thus reinforce this action by showing pleasure when the object is released. Encouraging your child to hand you a toy or a piece of food is another way to teach him how to open and close his hand. This can also be a valuable, early experience in sharing. Verbal cues such as "please give me," "thank you," "take it" should be used simultaneously with gestures to stimulate his use of language.

Once a child has learned to hold and to release, practice in throwing should begin. Most children start throwing without really being conscious of their action. The arm may be swung about and an object held in the hand released, landing to the surprise of the child on the floor. Somebody picks up the toy and hands it back to the child who now experiences pleasure in repeating the act. Throwing is a very rich learning experience for a child. Gross and fine movements of the upper limbs are involved and eye-hand coordination is established. Concepts of cause and effect and of basic spatial relationships may have their roots in such types of early play. Therefore, encourage your child to throw in preparation for more structured and complex ball play.

Parents of children with Down Syndrome are often concerned because objects may be thrown around indiscriminately. Your child may not be ready to distinguish what should and what should not be thrown. It will be up to you to remove breakable things until your child can differentiate between those appropriate for throwing and those that are "no-no's." If such situations are handled with effective and persistent discipline, then random throwing can be stopped without depriving a child of the opportunity to practice ball play. By now the child has probably progressed to the stage where he follows moving objects with interest, particularly when they move away or come closer. Perhaps he is ready to find out that an object that is "gone" is not gone forever.

The famous Swiss psychologist, Jean Piaget, has stressed the concept of permanence as an important stage of cognitive development. As a result, his ideas have lately been incorporated into various stimulation programs. The following are a few of the activities which can be used to acquaint your child with the permanence of objects.

1. Playing peek-a-boo: Cover the child's face with your hand or a cloth, disappear behind a door, some furniture, or curtains and then reappear; also put the child's own hands over his eyes in playing peek-a-boo.

2. Hide-and-seek games: Put your hand over a toy to hide it; put a coin in your child's fist and then turn his palm upside down to rediscover it; attach a toy to a string, let the toy drop over the edge of the table, then retrieve the toy by pulling the string; hide a toy under a pillow or box and show the child how to find it; roll a ball under a table or chair and let the child look for it.

A physical therapist, occupational therapist, or child development specialist may be of considerable help to you in providing suggestions for the correct choice and use of toys and other materials to enrich your child's learning experiences and improve his fine motor skills.

It is more important to observe and understand the way a young child manipulates objects and plays with them than to check developmental time schedules in order to find out how your child's performance rates in comparison to another individual or group of children. There are many diverse aspects of a child's play which influence his total performance; interest, dexterity, muscle strength, attention span, and experience are only a few of the many factors which make the outcome of an event a success or a failure. Consequently, your child's play should be evaluated carefully by a professional experienced in early child development, in order to help you to play effectively with your child.

Although the average child usually chooses materials suitable for a particular motor and cognitive developmental stage, children with Down Syndrome are known to pick less challenging toys and to continue playing with them beyond the time when they are ready to go on to more complex play activities. They frequently lack the initiative to explore new situations. If exposed to challenges they may at first show refusal and a great deal of frustration. With appropriate support and assistance, a mentally retarded child will become increasingly interested in more demanding tasks, as long as they are presented in a way that gives the child a feeling of enjoyment and success.

"Action toys" are preferable to those which may have some educational value but do not provide sufficient excitement and fun. Your child's attempts at playing should always result in some tangible and visible change brought about by his own effort. For instance, he pushes a button and a Jack jumps out of the box; he pushes down and a spinning top whirls; he opens an old pocketbook and lovely things are found there.

Generally, it is a good idea to present your child with only one or two toys at a given time. This will lead to a more thorough exploration and handling of toys than occurs in a situation where too many interesting things are introduced all at once. In the latter event a burden is placed on the child to make a decision for which he is most likely not yet ready. Usually, he will flit from one toy to another without benefiting very much from any of them. Many communities have recently developed "toy libraries" where parents can obtain age appropriate toys for their child. The toy librarians or child development specialists will be able to help parents to choose their desired playthings for their child.

There are few things which enchant a child as much as the discovery of a cabinet or a closet drawer. Provide such a place for your child, but combine it with a structured learning experience. Help him learn to remove only a few things at a time and to replace them before taking out new playthings. Help him share his treasures with siblings and friends, and to make some decisions and choices himself.

· Given other needs and demands, you may not have too much time to play with your child. Therefore, learn how to use your time most effectively. Sit down to play when your time and mind are really free, even if only for a short time. Devote the time you have to one play activity rather than to several. Analyze in as much detail as you can what it is you want your child to learn in a given situation. Break the activity down into many smaller parts. Ignore failures but praise successes, small as they may be. Use frequent repetitions, but stop before the child becomes bored with the activity. For a while, become a child yourself and share the joy of playing.

11

FEEDING
THE YOUNG CHILD
WITH DOWN SYNDROME

Elizabeth Zausmer and Siegfried M. Pueschel

Fortunately, most of the children with Down Syndrome do not have major feeding problems. The reflexes that involve sucking and swallowing are usually well developed at birth; as a matter of fact, they are present long before the baby is born. It is well known that the sucking and swallowing mechanisms involve structures of the mouth and throat including the tongue, palate, cheeks, and lips. A stimulus to the mouth such as touch or taste will elicit a sucking motion which is usually well coordinated with swallowing.

Some infants, however, may have initial difficulties with sucking, swallowing, and later with biting and chewing. These children will need some help and their parents will require special instructions in techniques of positioning and handling the child during feeding.

There are several reasons why some children with Down Syndrome may encounter these difficulties with feeding during the first few months of life:

1. Often there is decreased muscle strength of one or several structures of the mouth. Such muscle weakness may make it more difficult to move the food from the front to the back of the mouth or from one side to the other.

114

2. Some children tend to keep the mouth open which may further impede transporting food to the back of the mouth.

3. The roof of the mouth (palate) is usually narrow and shorter in length.

4. Another factor is related to the overall delay in development of the infant with Down Syndrome.

For these reasons parents may need advice and assistance from a pediatrician, a physical or occupational therapist, a nurse, nutritionist, or other professional in the field of child development who is knowledgeable in feeding problems of handicapped children.

After careful evaluation of the baby's feeding difficulties, the parents should be given instructions, demonstrations, and the opportunity of supervised practice in the various techniques that will help the child to obtain appropriate and effective patterns of sucking, swallowing, later chewing, and eventually self-feeding. Moreover, techniques in positioning and handling the infant during feeding, as well as the psychological and environmental aspects, will need to be discussed with the parents.

It is important that during feeding the infant be held in an upright or half upright position with his head well supported. Feeding an infant who is lying on his back or who is sitting with the head tilted backwards should be avoided since it might cause him to choke or to aspirate some of the milk. Also, propping the bottle or the use of a bottle holder is an undesirable practice. As a mother (or father) feeds her infant she usually enjoys holding the baby close to her, supporting the baby's head with her arms. Both mother and infant should be in a comfortable position.

We do not agree with some professionals who discourage mothers from breast feeding the infant with Down Syndrome. If the parents prefer breast feeding, if the infant is able to suck well, and if there are no medical contraindications, an infant with Down Syndrome can be breast fed as any other newborn.

If the baby is bottle fed, the bottle should be held in a position which allows the neck of the bottle to remain filled with milk or other liquids. Since a steady flow of milk makes sucking easier, one should prevent the nipple from collapsing. During feeding the infant should be permitted to burp several times. Then the parent might want to hold the baby upright against her shoulder or lean the baby slightly forward while sitting on her lap. If the baby's suck is weak or he tires easily during feeding, one might enlarge slightly the nipple hole so that the milk will flow easier. At times sucking can be stimulated by feeding in a circular motion occasionally pressing upward on the baby's palate and then down on his tongue. On occasion, a nipple for premature infants which is softer and longer may be used for babies with weak muscles. Sometimes, mothers might want to use a pacifier which will help to improve sucking by strengthening the muscles in the lips and cheeks. This also will encourage the infant to close his lips and to help retract the tongue. Gradually, the infant will overcome the feeding problem and the parents as well as the child will be more relaxed and will enjoy mealtimes together. After a few months, the child's hands can be placed on the bottle to encourage holding it.

If the child with Down Syndrome keeps his mouth open or his tongue protrudes during feeding, swallowing will be impaired. Since sucking and swallowing difficulties are often related, the above suggestions also will improve the baby's swallowing. Should swallowing difficulties continue, it is advisable to ask for professional assistance.

Usually between the second and fourth months, solid foods will be introduced in the baby's diet. Many infants with Down Syndrome do not have any difficulty taking solid foods from a spoon. Some babies, however, are unable to transfer the food to the back of the mouth. Often the tongue will push the food out. This can be helped by placing the spoon on the tongue with some downward pressure. By gently pressing downward on the infant's upper lip and holding the chin up, his mouth will be closed. Gradually, the infant will accept food offered by spoon and will learn to close his mouth spontaneously during feeding. The choice of the shape and the size of the spoon, the pressure and direction used for placement of the spoon into the child's mouth, as well as the volume and texture of the food, are important factors in the initial phase of spoon feeding.

Another important aspect of early feeding practices concerns finger-feeding. As the infant grows, he will grasp objects within his reach and bring them to his mouth to suck on and explore. A cookie or a biscuit can be placed in the child's hand which he might bring to his mouth for such oral exploration. Soon the infant will learn to use his hands to bring foods to his mouth. Crackers or dry cereals may also be offered to encourage grasping which initially might be done with the whole hand. Soon he will use the thumb and four fingers, and later when more mature, his thumb and forefinger will pick up interesting food objects to bring to his mouth.

Actually, exploration through vision, combined with the use of hands to bring objects to the mouth, is a rather complex motor act and requires that the baby has reached a certain developmental level. Some children with Down Syndrome might not engage in such activity and must be shown that the hand can be used to bring rewarding foods to the mouth. Parents should encourage the child to dip the fingers into foods, and then put the food into his mouth. In the beginning the parents will have to guide the child's hands through these movements by using food which is particularly appealing to the infant such as applesauce, whipped cream, or pudding. Soon the child will engage in such activities spontaneously. Many children with Down Syndrome use the fingers for eating considerably longer than do other children.

Once the child is ready and demonstrates the ability to pick up foods himself, various finger foods such as cooked vegetables, pieces of meat, and cheese can be offered during mealtime. The new experience of finger feeding can be educational and fun. The child will learn new shapes, colors, and textures.

Often parents are afraid that the child might choke on solid foods or they might think their baby will not be able to handle such finger foods when teeth have not erupted yet. It is important that such foods be offered to the young child since he gets used to the different textures and will use his gums, tongue, and jaws to start the chewing motion. Strained baby food should be discontinued when the infant is six to eight months old; junior and toddler foods, and later table foods, should be given instead.

During the second year of life most children with Down Syndrome can be taught to spoon feed themselves. In the beginning it may be necessary to guide the child's arm and hand repeatedly through the movements from plate to mouth and back to plate. Obviously, eating with a spoon demands a well coordinated sequence of varied skills, including stability of neck and shoulder muscles, adequate reach of arms, judgment of directions and distance from plate to mouth, correct grasp of the spoon handle, efficient swooping movements with the edge of the spoon, and the ability of bringing the spoon to the mouth. Gradually, less assistance will need to be provided and soon the baby will happily feed himself. Good results in self-feeding should always be acknowledged by the adult through encouraging words or a smile. The foundation of acquiring the important social skill of completely sharing a meal with other people must be laid in early childhood.

Children frequently make a greater effort to feed without assistance if they are allowed to have their meal at the dinner table with the rest of the family. The child should be placed in a comfortable position at a height where he can see what is going on around him. The food should be in a deep dish to avoid excessive spilling. A piece of plastic material or some paper might be placed on the floor so that the spilled food can be easily cleaned up after the meal. Initially, "messy" eating patterns have to be expected.

An exciting feeding experience will be the introduction of drinking from a cup. In the beginning the infant will spill liquids, but soon he will learn that the lips have to close around the rim of the cup to allow successful drinking. The child should be in an upright position when the cup with liquids is offered to him. Initially, thicker liquids such as frappes are easier to sip than thinner liquids. After the child has managed to drink from a cup, he can be gradually introduced to holding the cup by placing his hands around the cup and grasping the handles. Independent cup drinking will usually occur during the second year of life.

Undoubtedly, the nutritional value of certain foods will have to be taken into consideration. Adequate protein, fat, carbohydrates, and minerals, as well as sufficient vitamins, should be offered to the child according to his age. The quality and quantity of food should allow optimal growth and development. Yet, one should avoid overfeeding the child. Since some children with Down Syndrome tend to become overweight, attention should be paid to the proper nutritional intake of the child.

Although the rate of development of the child with Down Syndrome may be slower and he may have needs that require special understanding, most often the child will accomplish self-feeding and most feeding problems will be overcome in time.

==12

THE NURSERY SCHOOL YEARS

Claire D. Canning

Just as early intervention programs enhance the development of the child with Down Syndrome, nursery school also plays a very important role in his life. As parents, we ask ourselves, "Is there really a need to send a child whom we feel more protective of than we do of our other children away from the bosom of the home even for a few hours, at the tender age of three?" Having experienced these emotions, I feel, in retrospect, that nothing can replace a valuable nursery school experience.

We all want what will be best for our child and we realize that all children, even the most intelligent, have different needs. This becomes more complicated for the parents of a Down Syndrome child because we have no role models to follow or methods for training simple self-help skills that other children learn automatically. School becomes very important to the family because it extends the feeling of family and represents community support. Both a child and his family need the extra reinforcement that can come from school. It is a most appropriate adjunct to a family's daily efforts to care for its mentally handicapped child.

How do we prepare the child for nursery school? Since feelings of parental anxiety are so easily transmitted to the child, we should try very hard to overcome our own very normal anxieties to help ensure a smooth transition for our child. Public exposure is probably the best method of introducing a child with Down Syndrome to his community. Let him get to know strangers through everyday contacts. Take him to the supermarket, the zoo, church, anywhere you regularly go, to help your child feel comfortable in everyday situations. Tell your child, even if he cannot understand everything, that you are going to visit school with him.

We drove to school each day for a week, often just to walk around the building and yard. We spoke to the principal, met teachers, even boarded the school buses, so that when the day of parting arrived it would not be traumatic. We were fortunate to have a school bus driver who was one of the world's nicest men. For Martha, getting there was half the fun of the day. For very young or more handicapped children, an aide may ride on the bus to provide extra supervision and help if necessary. Some of the buses for special children have hydraulic lifts for wheelchairs and, of course, seat belts to ensure further safety. You may want to check these features yourself before your child starts school. Here too, we began to experience a beautiful feeling of community support. Excellent programs are available and many wonderful and qualified people really want to help.

What can the child with Down Syndrome learn in nursery school? So very many things! Just as our normal children have varying talents, three-year-old children with Down Syndrome will span a wide range of development. Each child, however, can profit from social interaction and gentle discipline, by working on self-help skills, by improving gross and fine motor coordination, and by learning to live with all types of behavior.

Learning to play is one of the most valuable skills a

child can acquire in nursery school. Play is a natural means of growth and learning. In the early stages, the child with Down Syndrome needs help in play. He must imitate, learn through doing, and make things happen. Even when limited in his ways, the child can feel, touch, taste, and smell. He must make choices and share. Limits are placed on his behavior, and he must learn to cooperate. All these skills help to shape positive behavior, and aid in implementing educational and parental goals.

It may seem trivial if one has not shared the early experiences of a child with Down Syndrome, but the accomplishment of toilet training seems like the greatest milestone of early nursery school experience. Recently, a legislator is said to have complained about the cost of programs for the handicapped, stating that for all the money spent, some children learned nothing all year but toilet training. Another more compassionate senator replied that if he thought about the most valuable skill he had learned in his lifetime, and had to choose between reading the classics or learning toilet training, he would instantly choose the latter. There is no further need to comment on what this means in all of our lives.

With new Federal legislation mandating the education of all handicapped children (P.L. 94–142) and with new directions required by society today, parents have many more choices for the education of children with Down Syndrome. You may choose for your child a regular or special nursery school, a private or publicly funded preschool for handicapped children. You should make your choice as objectively as possible depending on your child's level of functioning, and what seems like the best option in your community.

If you choose a regular nursery school, it should be small. To be effective, its teacher should have an interest in the special child, a healthy dose of compassion, and a sound general understanding of child development. Some parents send their child to a regular nursery school for three days, then to a special school for mentally handicapped children for two days. The main advantage of this arrangement seems to be a greater exposure to language from children who are more advanced in order to aid the child with Down Syndrome in language development. One parent has told us of sending his child to a special Sunday School class, then to a "normal" one. He discovered that the child was more interested and learned more in the latter.

We chose a diagnostic class in an integrated public school. This is a small heterogeneous group of children with a wide range of abilities. Eight children, three to six years old, are taught by a special education teacher and a full-time aide. The class includes culturally disadvantaged, learning-disabled, and mentally retarded children, grouped for the possibility of harmonizing diverse and conflicting potential learning problems. The smallness of the class gives the needed extra assurance of support. It stresses the importance of developing social competence. Receptive and expressive language development is emphasized, though lessons are geared to individual readiness in all skills. Speech and language therapy is given, physical therapy is provided if needed, and music, art, physical education, and library specialists all work together for the development of the child. A hot lunch (a great self-feeding skill help) is served, followed by a rest period. The teachers all exhibit great sensitivity which must be attributed to a happy combination of skill, compassion, and specialized training.

In whichever type of school you choose for your child, it is important that there be frequent interaction between nursery school personnel and parents. Parent participation should be welcomed and encouraged since it helps carry over school training into the home. In short, open communication is of vital importance to assure your child's optimal growth. Three to six are important years for the shaping of positive behavior. The good nursery school teacher knows how to approach each child including how to reinforce positive behavior. Parents, in turn, can continue this work in the home. There must be mutual respect and understanding of a variety of learning systems and options, with all working together toward the same goal, the growth of the handicapped child.

Are there any disadvantages to early schooling? The obvious one is exposure to other children. Because the child with Down Syndrome is usually more susceptible to respiratory infections, he may at first have more colds, and the inevitable childhood diseases. As times passes, however, his resistance becomes greater. We can all help very much if, when our child is sick, we use common sense and do not expose other children to his illness.

What do these nursery school years accomplish in maturation? They open new worlds for a Down Syndrome child and his family. They enable the child to participate in a broader world. For a mother, it is important to see her child function out of the home. Too close a relationship will not help either mother or child to function as independent individuals. The few hours taken up by the child's attendance at school in a well-chosen situation allows a mother time to perform other tasks or pursue her own interests. Mother and child can become better and stronger individuals for the time they spend away from each other. Then, refreshed, a mother can greet her child with renewed vigor, proudly inspecting the school papers and drawings that are so important to his sense of accomplishment.

The joy of discovery which is nurtured in nursery school is so important to the mentally handicapped child. Eventually, the child who seems to function best is the child who has been allowed to try and to grow. Your child is a unique human being. He should be given the opportunity to progress to the fullest realization of his human dignity.

=13

THE SCHOOL YEARS

Siegfried M. Pueschel

Entering School

Like any other child, the child with Down Syndrome is a product of genetic endowment, culture, and an environment shaped by people and events. Upon entering school he is still very much in the process of developing and growing with his own capacity for maturation and achievement. Beginning the school years will open up an entirely new world for most children with Down Syndrome; for some it might be just an extension of previous preschool experience.

In anticipation of school, parents can be of assistance in giving the child with Down Syndrome a good start. In the first few days, it is the responsibility of both parents and teachers to help the child adjust and settle in school. The success of their efforts will depend largely on the experiences the youngster has had at home in preschool years. The child who has been permitted to explore his world freely but safely, and has been able to broaden the scope of his activities, usually has little difficulty in making a happy adjustment from home to school. Encouraging his attempts at independence will prepare him for being away from home and mother for considerable parts of the day. If he has been allowed increasingly to do things for himself such as dressing, going to the bathroom, or managing his food at mealtimes, routines such as eating in the cafeteria and taking care of his own needs will not be a major problem.

If he has had an opportunity to play with other children he should find it relatively easy to interact with his classmates at school. If the child is used to contributing to the family's household tasks he will also be able to put toys away at school and help the teacher. If he has learned to listen and has been stimulated in language development, communication in school should not be a problem. The child who has been raised in an atmosphere which is neither overpermissive nor overprotective, but in which respect for each other's rights is the rule, should have little difficulty in accepting discipline in school.

To many parents' surprise, most children adjust well to school without major problems. At times, adjustment difficulties become apparent in the child who has had little exposure to the outside world, who has been reared in an overprotective home environment, and who has stayed too close to his mother during the first few years of life. A step-by-step adjustment from home to school is essential. Teacher and parents need to look for connecting links between the two environments as the child with Down Syndrome crosses the threshold into school life. Working together, parents and teachers can provide the security, comfort, and happiness in which a child can grow and learn.

Before the child with Down Syndrome begins his educational program, he should undergo an interdisciplinary evaluation. Such an assessment should focus on his physical abilities and needs, his intellectual development, his capacity to learn—including social and environmental aspects—and a variety of other factors.

Parents and teachers frequently ask, "Is the child ready to enter school? Does he bring with him all the important elements which make learning feasible? In terms of physical growth, visual and auditory perception, motor, and other organic functions, is he developmentally ready to enter school? Does he have the social ability and emotional fitness to relate successfully and independently with other people and with his environment? Is he intellectually able to gain understanding and utilize information in everyday experiences? And with regard to language, is he able to communicate coherently with others?"

While these questions might well be appropriate concerning the "normal" child, we have to ask whether they also apply to the child with Down Syndrome. Perhaps the real question should not be, "Is the child ready for school?" but rather, "Is the school ready for the child?" Since many of the developmental functions one ordinarily expects of the "normal" child are not usually observed in the child with Down Syndrome, when he enters school, the educational program will have to be adapted to his ability and special needs. Therefore, we do have to ask, "Does the school provide all the elements necessary to meet the challenge of educating a youngster with Down Syndrome? Is the teacher ready to learn about the child's problem in order to help him most effectively? Will the educational program assist the student in preparation for life?"

When the child with Down Syndrome enters school, we often wonder what he will get out of the educational experience. Surely, we hope that school provides the kind of stimulating and rich experiences in which the world appears as an interesting place to explore. Learning situations at school should help a child with Down Syndrome obtain a feeling of personal identity, self-respect, and enjoyment. They should give him an opportunity to engage in sharing relationships with others and prepare him so that he can later contribute productively to society. Schools should give a foundation for life by encouraging the development of basic academic skills, physical abilities, self-help skills, and social as well as language competence.

Some parents think that the school is supposed to teach only reading, writing, and arithmetic. While children with Down Syndrome are in need of these basic academic instructions, a good educational program, however, should also prepare a child for all areas of life. Things like getting a job done when it's supposed to be done, getting along well with people, and knowing where to go to find an answer are perhaps more important than the three R's.

What kind of learning should be provided during this period of development when the goal is to help the child with Down Syndrome gain a knowledge of the world that is meaningful to him? If the school approaches his education in terms of humanizing the teaching process, viewing each student as a person with an individual integrity all his own, exposing him to forces that will contribute to self-fulfillment in the broader sense, then the child with Down Syndrome will be given the opportunity to develop optimally in the educational setting. The true humanistic ideal that a man selects and creates a destiny for himself as an outgrowth of his education will need to be altered in some ways to be adapted to the individual capabilities and limitations of each person with Down Syndrome.

Educational Strategies

A child's immediate environment in school is an important factor in the educational process. It should provide physical, intellectual, and social stimulation. Ideally, the school environment should be structured so that each child has access to space, equipment, and materials necessary for his growth and development. Sometimes children with mental retardation are taught in poorly equipped, old school buildings. If inappropriate local circumstances prevail, children will suffer—they will not be allowed to grow physically and intellectually because of restrictions in the environment. Children need a stimulating classroom with ample space. Outdoor facilities should encourage motor activities that enable children to gain control of their bodies and develop greater coordination.

Children express thoughts and feelings through the use of their bodies, and space makes it possible for them to learn through experimentation. Thus, they can react to the world about them and use emotions as a means of communication in expressing their innermost thoughts and feelings. Since movement is such a prime factor for mentally retarded youngsters and since they should have extended opportunity to explore the physical world around them, they indeed need open space and appropriate equipment. A jungle gym, balancing beam, slides, wagons, and other play things will let them engage in appropriate motor activities. It is the way in which a child spontaneously manuevers with such objects that he learns to use his own body, and to appreciate both what he is and what he can do. A child needs the opportunity to begin to use himself as a physical organism with control and coordination, and to know himself as a person who has these skills.

At the same time, the child with Down Syndrome has a chance to learn what the nature of the physical world is all about. The things he sees around him exhibit both size and weight; the size and weight are impressions that register with him. The things he pushes around have certain built-in relations to other objects in a physical universe. He experiences pressure, leverage, balancing, and hoisting. Watching him we see lots of things: the child is learning and he is having fun. He is enjoying an activity he has planned and carried through by himself. It is this sense of accomplishment we seek to provide for children through various different aspects in his learning experience. We believe that each accomplishment, each skill, each mastery, adds an ingredient of belief in self and pleasure with what one is able to do in one's environment.

Children learn about space when they crawl under the table or stand on top of it. When they climb, run, jump, roll, skip, swing, and crawl, children get a feeling for height, distance, and speed. There must be open spaces where they can let their bodies stretch and move freely and narrow spaces where they must squeeze their bodies as tight as they can.

Children need to become familiar with the wider space around them. Many young children go directly from their homes to the bus and straight into the school without any idea of the distance involved or any landmark along the way. Walks around the neighborhood help to give children a sense of direction and distance. When children do not live too far from their school, one child at a time can lead his classmates to his house and thus show the way. It is important that the child with Down Syndrome learns the address and telephone number of where he lives and where to turn for help if he gets lost.

Although the concept of time is often difficult for young children with Down Syndrome to comprehend, they will soon begin to understand not only the length of time, but words such as after, before, tomorrow, this morning, and yesterday. During the early school years, they might not learn how to read a clock, but later they should be instructed how to tell time.

Learning seasons and special days help children with Down Syndrome develop a calendar-time concept. They learn that in winter it is often too cold to play outdoors, yet in summer they are allowed to get wet under the sprinkler. They need to know what to expect in each season and how it may effect their lives. Some teachers hang up large calendars in their classrooms giving the names and dates of each day in the month. Every morning teacher and children repeat both the day and date. They talk about what will happen that day or what is ahead tomorrow. In this way children learn the names of the days and months. At the same time they experience how one day is different from another. They see that Saturdays and Sundays are not the same as other days because they don't go to school on those days. The weather also sets one day apart from the next which suggests that a teacher might use the calendar to record the weather. If the day is sunny, a child might want to color a sun in that day's space. Or if it is rainy, another child might want to draw some raindrops. Gradually, children will get a feel for time concepts and learn the meaning of time.

Birthdays are very special days for children. Most teachers are careful to remember each child's birthday by singing "Happy Birthday," by having a birthday cake for him, and by giving the child a gift to take home. A teacher might write his students' birthdays on the calendar so that each child can see how soon his birthday will come. Children enjoy the attention they get on their birthdays.

The major holidays are usually celebrated in schools and children are often making special things: at Halloween they might make a paper bag mask; at Christmas, trim a tree; and at Easter, dye eggs. A lot of things can be learned by becoming involved in these activities. If a teacher can tell stories about why people wear masks, or how the custom of trimming the tree came about, or what the meaning is for dyeing Easter eggs, then the children will learn about their heritage, historical events, and certain customs. Many holiday activities provide a good learning experience for the child and at the same time are happy events to be remembered.

Children have to become increasingly sensitive to the world in which they live. To observe keenly what is around them, they have to open their eyes and ears to their surroundings. Partly, this is done inside school where many different kinds of materials are provided for play and manipulation. These materials have many uses in children's play. They include a house in a corner of the classroom, letter blocks to build with, paints and easels, the storybooks on the table, and the puzzle boards on the shelf. But just play things of course, never perform the real magic of learning. The magic ultimately comes from the teacher and all those involved in a child's education. Thus, the child who becomes keenly aware of what is happening around him is also building up a feeling of belonging to the world in which he lives.

Furthermore, we want to provide children with Down Syndrome the opportunity for acquiring a large repertoire of what we might call action responses—school life for the child with retardation consists of this kind of experience. For example, with blocks, when a child builds certain structures, he is learning how to make objects follow his intentions. In general, what is important here is to give a child the opportunity to develop manipulative, constructive skills and with these skills to have the experience of changing things in this world. The child is satisfying a basic need to impress himself upon the world around him. And, at the same time, he acquires knowledge and understanding of himself as someone who can change his environment in a constructive and positive way.

Another kind of experience for learning takes us into an area where the child can produce his own particular view of things based on experiences that have been meaningful for him. In his gestures he is producing actions he has seen. In his paintings, drawings, and modelings with clay, he is trying to bring back experiences he has had. We should provide a child with multiple materials for his reliving of his experiences. Paint, clay, and music to which he moves symbolically are all vehicles for helping the child deepen and select meanings important to him in reliving his experience. If there is any way of gaining knowledge particularly suitable to this stage of development, it is in the dramatic play that children spontaneously devise, which nevertheless needs an attentive and understanding teacher for its support and encouragement.

In teaching the young child with Down Syndrome, a teacher will have to work at various levels of difficulties at different times. The teacher will be advised to use lots of examples in the process of explaining certain concepts. Repetition is crucial in the learning process of the child. Children like to sing the same songs over and over again. They enjoy doing the same puzzles and playing with the same toys. Just as it is important to introduce new things for children, one should also emphasize repeating activities that give pleasure and augment learning. The more children know about a particular subject, the more familiar they become with it, the better and more secure they feel, and the more fun they have.

For example, a teacher took her children to visit a fire station where they saw many new things. She knew that the children most likely would forget much of what they had seen and experienced. The next day she showed them a book about a fire station. The children pointed out how the fire engine in the book was different from the one they had seen. They were astonished that the firemen in the book had the same kind of dog they had seen at the fire station. A week later the teacher showed them some photographs she had taken at the fire station and again the children remembered their experiences with the help of these pictures. When the teacher arranged another visit at the fire station, the children were much more familiar with the surroundings and with the activities that took place there. Many knew their way around and recalled the different activities at the station. So, by repetition they gained from this learning experience.

The skillful teacher realizes that no amount of talking or reading or writing is as effective in teaching as it is for the child to feel a tangible object or to participate in a situation. Watching snow flakes gently coming down from the sky or to see rain spatter against the window is infinitely more meaningful to the child than seeing a picture in a book or even having another adult tell him about it. Real life situations can be more creative learning experiences. Opportunities for field trips provide the child with Down Syndrome a chance to learn how to live in a community with other people. Expeditions to zoos and parks let him see real life animals, trees and plants, and let him view the beauty of nature. Watching the mailman and policeman at work and interacting with them is a much more sustaining experience for the child with Down Syndrome than abstract presentations or even pictures in books.

One of the most important aspects of learning at all ages is that of motivation. Actually little or no learning takes place unless a person is motivated. Almost all children are curious and have a desire to learn. One should understand, however, that what may motivate or interest one person may fail to influence another.

It is most important that a child be put into a situation where he can achieve in the education process. Each child has his own potential which must be explored, evaluated, and then worked with. Achievement will give the child a good feeling. It will encourage him, raise his self-esteem, and lead to new endeavors. Often the right incentive can be a determining influence on the degree of effort put forth in accomplishing a task. A smile, an approving nod, a few words of praise, are usually enough to make a child with Down Syndrome try harder. A child thrives on an adult's approval. If the person working with a child is able to initiate a positive approach that the child can accept, effective guidance and learning will follow. But if the child feels that he is not accepted or that a person does not want to work with him, there will be a wall between teacher and student that will interfere with the learning process. In contrast, if a closeness exists between teacher and child, and if a kind approach is accompanied by smiles and verbal praise, the child will be encouraged, his inner drive will come to the surface, and he will be motivated to work. Children learn best when they are happy, when they can do things well, when they know what we want, and when we let them know we like what they do.

When one observes a good special education program, there are so many activities that go on all at once that it is sometimes hard to pinpoint exactly what each child is learning. A visitor, for instance, may find one child playing with a fire engine wearing a fireman's hat, two other children talking on a toy telephone, the next one pouring water from a pitcher into a cup, while another child tickles a hamster through the wire mesh of a cage. One might think, "What a confused place this! How can children learn when they are so scattered around?" Yet, these children are all learning in one way or another. For sure, they are not formally sitting in one row reciting the alphabet, but they are free to move about and work on independent projects, and thus learn much more about their world. The children who are scattered into many activities are following their own individual interests, and in the process they are learning about many aspects of life. Life is so complex that children have to try out many different things in order to make new learning a part of themselves.

While it is important to study the way children learn and what the needs for skillful and sensitive teaching are during this stage of development, attention should also be given to the fact that much depends on the way in which a teacher can relate to a child. It is essential that the child can trust the teacher. A great deal also depends on the extent to which a teacher can think along with a Down Syndrome child. The teacher should not expect him to be as reasonable or as logical as other children might be, but recognize him as an individual in his own way.

As a result of his school experience, a child with Down Syndrome should begin to see himself as a person who is capable of doing things, seeing things, and mastering things, who can communicate with adults and with other children, and who can enjoy his own ability to initiate activities and play.

Arts and Activities

All children, including the child with Down Syndrome, grow and develop physically and mentally. There are many different ways one can help strengthen their minds as well as their muscles, and teaching arts and crafts is one of them.

Most children love to make things. Too often, however, the handicapped child finds that there are many things he cannot do; hence, he may feel defeated before he even starts. Yet, we know from experience that he can make something out of wood or clay or use a paint brush. It might be primitive and perhaps unrecognizable, but it is a product that he has made himself. He has proven that he can do something. With the simplest of arts and crafts in a modest school or home environment, a child's development can be stimulated and enhanced. Materials and activities should be chosen carefully to make the greatest use of your child's ability.

Arts and activities can help your child acquire manual dexterity, eye-hand coordination, and social awareness. Such activities encourage a child to work and share with others. While he may want his own pair of scissors or box of crayons, he learns to share when there is only one pair of scissors available for three students. Your child will also develop a respect for the other person's property. He will learn not to destroy what the other person is doing. He will be taught good work habits, which include being tidy about himself and his work. Furthermore, the child will learn to follow instructions and carry a job through to completion. The child can be taught to do his best at all times and, even if his best is not up to what others are doing, it is still very acceptable.

Becoming involved in arts and crafts, the child can see a return for his efforts. When working with wood, paint, or completing a rug, he will see change taking place, and he knows that what he is doing is permanent. Art and craft objects can be put out for display, enabling children to gain recognition. Finally, they can take their work home, show it to family members, and can be proud of their accomplishments.

Arts and crafts activities also prepare the youngster with Down Syndrome for his future in that they help him acquire the mental discipline and job skills he will need for late vocational adjustment. Through involvement with arts and crafts, one may find out what kind of skills and talents a student has to help him in future working situations. Success in workshop jobs and in other work opportunities will depend upon judgment of color, shape, size, and weight. Knowing how to handle tools and materials at any level greatly increases your youngster's chance to become involved in productive work later.

Music and Rhythmic Activities

The child with Down Syndrome ordinarily loves music. Often, he responds more readily to music than to other activities in school. Music provides a gratifying experience and usually brings forth positive feelings in the child. Music can provide a feeling of participation and achievement, an acceptable outlet for physical and emotional tension, as well as considerable fun and happiness. Social development, group participation, following directions, and sharing and taking turns, can all be encouraged by getting a child with Down Syndrome involved in music.

Important use of music can be made in the areas of language development, auditory discrimination, and memory. Since language deficits and speech problems are usually present in the child with Down Syndrome, he can frequently communicate more easily through music than through verbalization. The practice of making speech sounds by associating sounds with actions and directions can reinforce many concepts and aid in the learning process. Music also plays a major role in developing a sense of rhythm and tempo. It aids coordination by encouraging the use of larger and smaller muscles in a controlled manner.

Through music, many children who exhibit abnormal behaviors become more relaxed, attentive, and motivated. Music encourages motivation for group participation as well as individual responses. The group involvement is important because many future life experiences depend on whether or not individuals can identify themselves comfortably in group situations.

Speech and Language

We interact with people in society primarily through communication and language. Communication is a particularly important aspect in the educational program for the child with Down Syndrome, for it is the key that unlocks the door to social adjustment. It involves more than simply the verbal or written message. Communication includes the ability to express feelings and thoughts, whether conveyed by gestures, expressions, or words. The use of words becomes a major tool for a child in dealing symbolically with his experiences and in being able to think in more complicated ways, for it is through language that we learn of our world and share our experiences with others.

The development of language and concepts helps a child to organize his ideas about the meaning of things in the world in which he lives. Objects are not only objects; they are things which can be manipulated and which have names. They have functions, shapes, colors and sizes, and they are related to each other. All of these aspects can be put into words.

In order to foster language development, clear speech,

expansion of vocabulary, and good speaking habits, it is essential that children be required to speak in a loud and clear voice. In addition, the child should learn to speak slowly and understandably.

To encourage language and speech development, one should assess at what level a child with Down Syndrome is functioning, what his strengths and weaknesses are. One will also have to study the environmental situation, the child's emotional stability, and his ability to hear adequately.

The child's hearing ability is of great significance. In recent years, due to new assessment techniques, the hearing of children with Down Syndrome has often been found defective. Because of the somewhat different anatomical structures within his hearing apparatus and the frequent upper respiratory infections, the child with Down Syndrome often develops ear infections. Subsequently, fluid accumulation in the middle ear is noted. These problems commonly lead to mild or moderate conductive hearing deficits. While some professionals do not consider these minor hearing problems important, studies have shown that even mild hearing deficits may have detrimental influences upon language development and speech. Upon entering school, all children should have a hearing evaluation; but it is particularly needed for children who have experienced upper respiratory and ear infections, and who respond inappropriately when approached verbally.

The majority of children with Down Syndrome will benefit from speech and language therapy. They are seldom helped, however, by short-term therapeutic interventions. In order to facilitate his communicative skills, a child with Down Syndrome will need regular assistance in the area of speech and language through his school years. The primary goal of such intervention is to help children develop adequate speech and language as early as possible, to look for specific disabilities, to determine the degree of deficit present in the child, and to explore the avenues considered best for reaching the child.

The therapeutic approach to children with Down Syndrome who have delayed speech and language development should be carried out quietly, surely, and warmly. Speech and language therapy should start with activities appropriate to the level at which a child is presently operating. If the therapist begins with some activities the child can do with ease, the child will feel more comfortable and adjust better to the new task at hand. Therapy also becomes more cohesive if the therapist plans some activities that can be continued by the teacher and by the parents at home. The therapist should make the sessions as pleasureful as possible and let the child know that he is indeed accomplishing a great deal.

Speech and language therapy might be carried out in a hospital or a center specializing in children with handicapping conditions. Speech therapists are usually aware of the speech and language difficulties associated with Down Syndrome. More convenient, and sometimes more effective, therapy might be provided within the school setting where a natural carry-over into the classroom situation is possible. Ideally, a speech and language therapist should interact with a child on a daily basis. In situations involving a personnel shortage, a therapist might only see a child with Down Syndrome for a ten-minute period once a week or be forced to give speech therapy in group sessions. It is important that speech and language therapy be provided according to a child's need. We do not agree with some professionals who feel that speech therapy for mentally retarded children is a waste of time. It has been demonstrated that children with Down Syndrome will gain from an appropriate approach to speech and language therapy, and that their cognitive abilities, their emotional stability, and their outlook on life will benefit from such intervention.

Integration or Segregation

Although the question of whether or not to separate retarded children from normal children in schools has been discussed extensively during the past decade, it still remains a controversial issue. There is no clear-cut answer to the question of whether children with Down Syndrome should be educated together with other retarded children in special education classes, or intermixed with nonhandicapped children. If children with Down Syndrome are separated from children in regular schools, the question then arises whether they should be placed in a class for trainable or educable mentally retarded children.

Traditionally, educators have differentiated between educable and trainable retarded children. The former group of children is said to profit from academic instructions, i.e., they can be taught reading, writing, and arithmetic. Since trainable children are thought to lack these academic abilities, emphasis in the classroom has been on teaching social and self-help skills. Often, the placement into one class or the other has been made quite arbitrarily, depending on the local definition of educable and trainable.

Too often in the past, the child with Down Syndrome has been routinely considered either moderately or severely retarded and, without assessing his individual abilities, he was placed into a class for trainable retarded youngsters. Such an unreasonable decision does not take into account the child's strengths in certain areas of development.

We feel that any child, including the child with Down Syndrome, is in need of both training and education. This means that a child with Down Syndrome will need instruction in basic academic subjects as well as training in social and self-help skills so important for daily living. Moreover, recent advances in teaching methods and novel educational strategies for children with special needs do not justify a clear-cut division between educable and trainable children.

According to the proponents of such programs, children in self-contained classrooms, excluded from the mainstream of childhood education, have less fear of failure and a greater opportunity to excel than retarded children in regular classes. Some authorities feel that it is better to place a child with Down Syndrome in a situation where he has a chance to succeed, where the work is adapted to his limitations and his handicaps, and where success follows a reasonable expenditure of effort. In such an environment, there will be less competition and the child with special needs will not be overlooked or pushed aside as might happen in a larger classroom with "normal" children. Arguments favoring the self-contained class emphasize that the special education teacher is thoroughly prepared and trained and fully understands the needs and nature of the retarded child. Segregation also facilitates a more homogeneous grouping of students with similar disabilities and needs. Moreover, the child with Down Syndrome will often benefit from individual or small group instruction. Therefore, many educators support segregation, indicating that the social adjustment of the child with Down Syndrome, like other children with retardations, may exceed that of retarded children educated in regular classrooms.

On the other hand, proponents for integration in regular classes argue that the segregation of children in specifically labeled groups may create exactly the kind of damage to the self-esteem of those children that one wishes to avoid. Integration is supposed to improve a student's self-image by not stigmatizing him as being special or different. Integration proponents say that freely mixing children of all sorts provides a realistic environment in which the handicapped child can best learn what he can and what he cannot do and how to cope with evolving problems. While teasing will occasionally occur in the integrated class, it will be less damaging psychologically than segregation.

The presence of handicapped children in regular classes will also be helpful to nonhandicapped children. They will acquire a better understanding of and a greater respect for individual differences. These "normal" children need to know about the existence of handicaps. They need to learn how to deal with children with Down Syndrome without becoming contemptuous or over solicitous since they will share life in the community with handicapped persons in the future.

Whether or not to integrate the child with Down Syndrome depends primarily on your goals and educational purpose. It should be realized that in preparing your child for his future, education must concern itself with what goes on in the mind of the child rather than what goes on in a classroom. Redefinition of goals, academic progress, learning profiles, learning characteristics, and anticipated

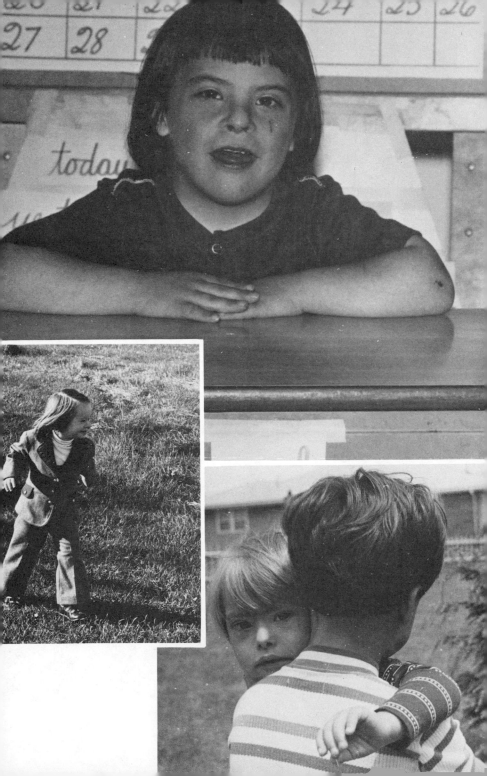

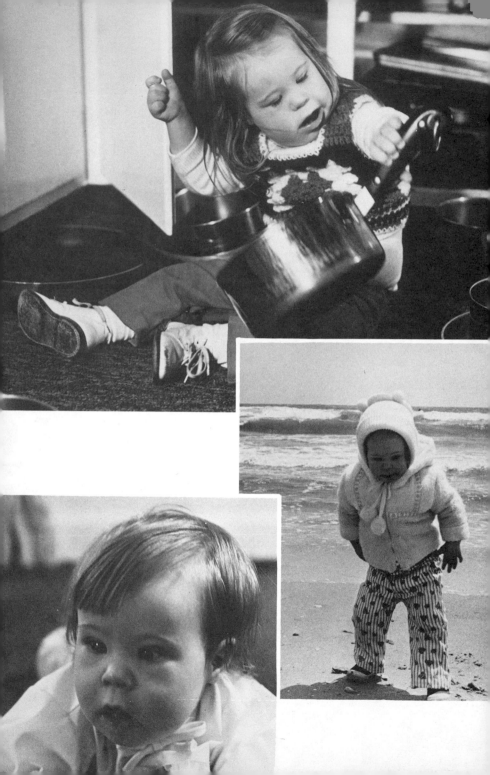

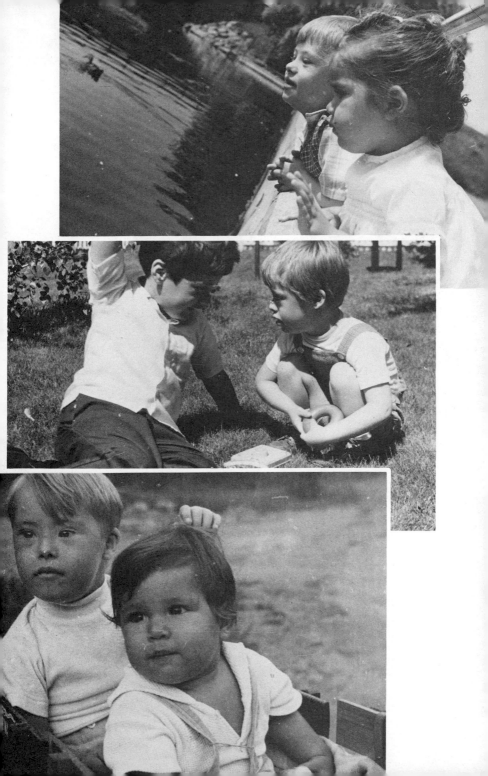

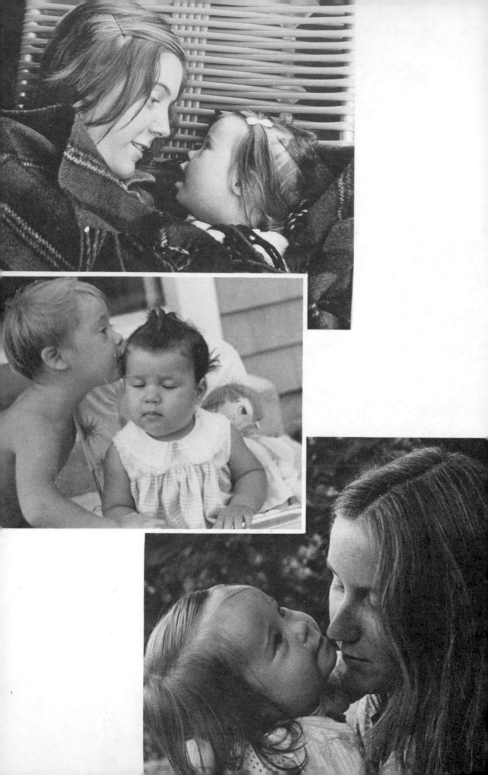

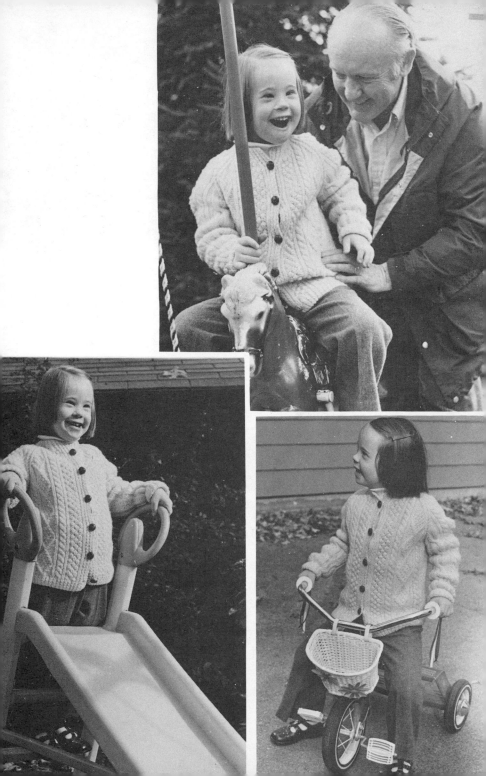

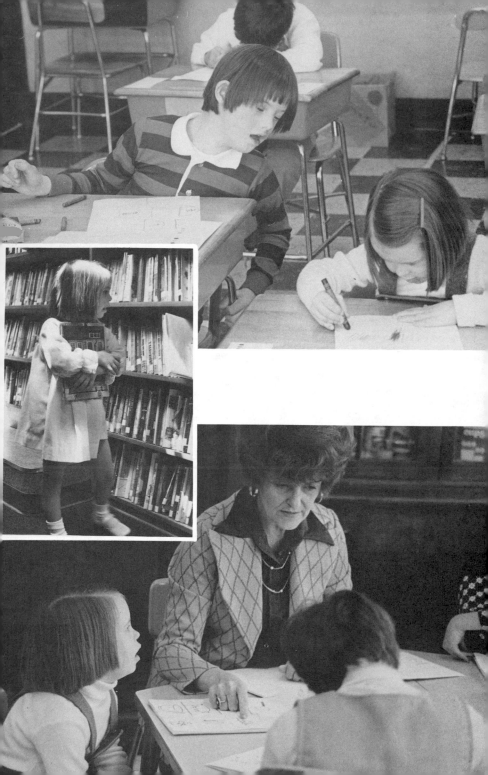

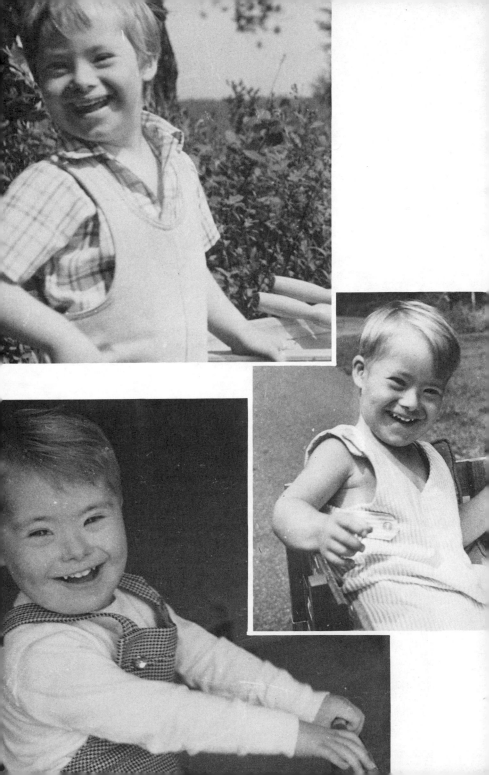

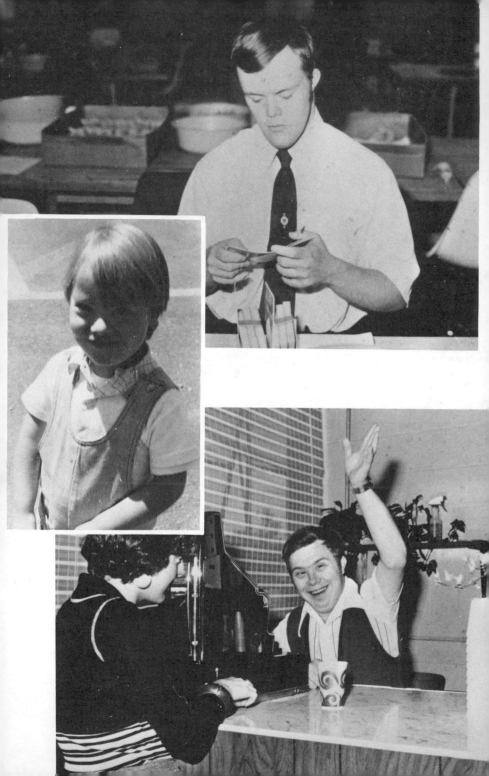

future life achievements are important elements which need to be considered when the question of his placement in a regular or segregated special classroom arises. Other factors which enter into the discussion are your child's emotional stability, his social function, intellectual abilities, the quality of each particular classroom, and local attitudes towards the child with Down Syndrome.

If the school is to prepare children for life and provide them with the knowledge and tools to help them function optimally in society, then these children will have to be exposed to normal children. Some form of integration is not only desirable, but necessary. In certain academic subjects, however, segregation might be called for. Such intermediate strategies (partly segregated, partly integrated) are gaining acceptance. In general, they consist of operating special classes within a regular public school where the retarded student attends special classes for certain subjects and is integrated into normal classes for other subjects, like physical education and arts and crafts.

HOME AND COMMUNITY AS A SOURCE OF ENRICHMENT

Siegfried M. Pueschel

Even when he is attending school, the child with Down Syndrome spends much of his time in the home environment. There is at least an hour in the morning while he gets ready for school, several hours in the afternoon when he enjoys playtime, and more hours in the evening when he can have fun with other members of his family. There is even more time available during weekends, holidays, and vacations. The child actually spends more time at home than at school.

Obviously learning does not only happen in school; a great deal of learning occurs in the home or when crossing the street, or playing with a friend. There are so many experiences to become involved in and new things to be investigated in both home and neighborhood. The process of learning will be accentuated when loving and understanding family members help a child with Down Syndrome achieve his maximum potential.

The child with Down Syndrome can benefit from a variety of experiences in the home relating to many areas of development. Particularly in the area of language development, much can be accomplished. The way a parent talks with a child, explaining certain activities and events or reading stories, will undoubtedly stimulate a child's language development.

Exploring the world beyond the school can be an exciting learning experience. Walking in the neighborhood or driving down a road, children will learn about traffic. They will have to learn the dangers involved in being out on the street, that traffic lights turning red mean STOP, and that green means GO. While children often know what the red, yellow, and green traffic lights mean, they also have to know what motions a policeman or school patrol uses to signal them to STOP or GO. Simple games with one child acting as policeman or directing traffic, either with a whistle, hand motions, or red and green paper signals, can help your children fix these signals firmly in their minds.

Since crossing the street can be dangerous, your child needs to be instructed to look out for hazards. He will need to know when, where, and how to cross the street. He has to be taught to look in both directions before crossing, and learn that certain striped areas tell us where to cross the streets more safely. He needs to know that he cannot run diagonally across a street without looking left and right. The dangers of traffic both on city streets and on rural highways makes it vital that he learn to understand traffic symbols at an early age.

While in the street, children may notice streetcars or big buses. They will have to learn about both because one day they might want to go to work by public transportation. While entering the bus they will have to be polite, to let some people go first or help others who have difficulties climbing. They will also have to know how to give the conductor the correct amount of money to cover the fare. Many things can be learned on the bus, including how to behave in public and how to get around in the city. Going on a streetcar or train can be lots of fun for children. They will experience and see many new things. They might learn what a bridge is and what tunnels are for, while simultaneously discovering a new world as they observe the hectic city life.

After school there should be recreation. Yet a good recreation program for children with Down Syndrome takes imagination, resourcefulness, and plain hard work. Often, it is a bigger task than one family can handle alone; it has to be the concern of the local community. Some children might love music, but others prefer swimming, crafts, or artwork. The retarded child should not be turned down or left out because of his limited intellectual endowment. Preferably. he should be integrated in recreational programs with other children. When this is not feasible, there should be special programs for children with handicapping conditions.

Boy and Girl Scouts programs have been successful with retarded children. Often in the younger age group of Cub Scouts and Brownies, it has been mentioned how much these boys and girls can accomplish together. Belonging to a group, wearing a uniform, and having the opportunity for personal achievement is as meaningful to the child with Down Syndrome as it is to other children. At times, parents have to organize themselves and secure the interest of a trained leader. Community centers, church groups, and YMCA's often provide recreational activities for retarded youngsters.

Camping is a particularly important experience for retarded children. Camp life emphasizes an atmosphere of relaxation and a freedom to explore, to enjoy sand, water, leaves, bugs, wind, and sky. It provides time to develop friendships and to train muscles and senses. Some children with Down Syndrome fit well into a camp with other children. Others might feel better when they attend camps for handicapped children. These camps should offer children pleasure away from home, a joy of nature, and the company of many new friends.

Parents also can help the child with Down Syndrome with his emotional needs. Like any child, he needs love, attention, and acceptance. He is in need of an environment in which he can grow up securely, where he can develop self-esteem and independence. If a child feels good about himself, if he has self-confidence, and if he can experience success, however small and insignificant it may seem, it will be very important for the child and his self-image. If parents have a positive perception of their child, it will be sensed by him, and he will feel loved and accepted. Emotional well-being is of utmost importance in the development of any child, but even more so for the retarded child.

As parents we often like to do things for our children. Yet, the development of independence is another salient feature in the maturational process of the child with Down Syndrome. It is important in the development of the child's self-esteem to feel satisfaction and accomplishment when he does something by himself. Therefore we might want to construct situations which are not too difficult, but which make it possible for a child to achieve success. Complicated situations only lead to frustrations, tempers, and stubbornness while a simple task might be mastered after he has been instructed how to do it. Sometimes it will take many repetitious attempts and patient encouragement, but finally, when a task has been accomplished a child will feel extreme satisfaction.

Parents often ask questions about discipline. Generally speaking, discipline should be a part of the normal life of any child. It is important, however, that discipline be applied gently and consistently in both home and school so that a child with Down Syndrome understands that both environments have the same standards. Since a child's social behavior is important in determining his chances in life, the pattern of discipline in the child with Down Syndrome will be significant. The child's appropriate social behavior is directly related to his acceptance in society and future vocational success. The child learns of responsibility and develops a sense of order when limits are established and standards are set.

The care of a child's clothing, dressing, and undressing are important aspects of his training. Because of the time it takes for a child to dress and undress, parents often take over and do it for the child. Most children entering school, however, are able to take off their clothes, hang up their coats, and zip their pants. Parents should encourage these activities and take pride in the child who is dressing himself.

A great deal of learning takes place when a child is allowed to handle his own clothes. Having a place of his own to keep his clothes will give him much pleasure. He can learn about order in placing his clothes in a drawer or in a closet space. Hooks should be low enough for him to be able to hang up his own clothes. Clothing does not need to be expensive, but much thought should be given to the attractiveness and comfortableness of clothing for a child with Down Syndrome. We should listen to a child's wishes and desires when we buy clothes for him. A child will often develop a sense of pride when he can choose his own clothing and dress himself neatly. A child should become aware that those who are observing him are proud of the way he looks and is dressed. Calling the child's attention to the neat appearance of others and acquainting him with standards of dress help him to develop self-awareness. Retarded children are much better accepted in society when they conform with general standards of cleanliness and wear proper attire.

Children need to be instructed in daily teeth brushing, also cleaning their shoes, washing their hands, and combing or brushing their hair. Grooming, appropriate haircuts, and neat clothing will help a child gain social acceptance.

During the first few years of life your child will have accomplished certain feeding skills and will have been taught self-feeding successfully. Some children still might have difficulties in manipulating a knife and fork and may need some help. Pouring milk, drinking from a cup without spilling, and managing knife and fork are important learning experiences that will improve a child's dexterity. During mealtimes, acceptable table manners and appropriate eating behaviors can be taught. When a child can experience mealtimes as enjoyable get-togethers, he gains a feeling of security.

The diet should be nutritious. It should contain enough protein for growth as well as the required carbohydrates, fats, and minerals needed at his age. Since some children with Down Syndrome tend to become overweight, you should not overfeed your child. It is a fact of life that our society accepts good looking, slim individuals more readily than slow moving overweight persons. Once children are used to eating a lot, they will continue to do so. They might learn that increased food intake can give them some satisfaction when they don't find accomplishments in other areas of life. Once a child is too heavy, he will move around less and may stop participating in regular family and school activities.

Eating out in a restaurant is another occasion at which a child with Down Syndrome can learn about social behaviors. The child will have to be prepared for these occasions. If family members give good examples, the child will follow suit and imitate such behavior. Usually, children with Down Syndrome have good table manners if a pattern is set for them.

To live in society, the child with Down Syndrome will have to achieve a degree of competence in social living. He must learn how to behave in the outside world and how to relate to people. He must learn to respect the rights and property of others and to tolerate behaviors of others in family, neighborhood, and community. If he knows how to behave in society, others will feel comfortable in relating to him. Children with Down Syndrome usually do not have difficulties relating to people in a friendly and outgoing fashion. Sometimes they might be too cordial. While it may be all right for a toddler to hug a stranger, such behavior is not accepted if done by an adolescent with Down Syndrome. Teaching a child with Down Syndrome appropriate social behaviors will make his life more enjoyable and increase the chances that he will be accepted in the community.

Neighbors play an important part in the child's efforts to socialize in the community. Parents do not have to feel ashamed to introduce a child with Down Syndrome to neighbors. When parents transmit their own pride in having this child, their neighbors will look upon the child in the same way. A child with Down Syndrome should be taught to greet neighbors politely and cheerfully. He also should be taught that we can help our neighbors.

Although socializing is an important aspect in the child's life, he should also learn to be alone some of his day and be able to entertain himself. Quiet times are growing times as well. It is at such times that a child may assimilate ideas he has gained and try out new things for himself. The child should have appropriate toys and materials to use so that quiet periods will not be boring for him or lead to self-stimulating behaviors. We all need time to ourselves and the child with Down Syndrome is no exception. We should respect his desire to be by himself and not interpret it as withdrawing or antisocial behavior.

As we have illustrated there are many experiences beyond the school environment which will help the child to prepare for life. Going shopping, visiting the library, calling at the home of friends, or going on picnics are exciting events that can foster social development, while exposing your child to new circumstances in the life of your community.

15⚌

SPECIAL CONCERNS IN ADOLESCENCE

Siegfried M. Pueschel

Adolescence is frequently a challenging time in life for both the young person and his family. It is a difficult period of transition for the adolescent who is attempting to free himself from the role of a child, but who is not yet fully equipped to assume the responsibility of adulthood. While this may be a very troublesome time for those of normal intellectual abilities, a retarded adolescent's problems are frequently intensified. Many retarded adolescents have the physical attributes of normal youngsters, yet they often do not possess the capabilities to cope with either the demands of their environment or their own desires for independence. They are faced with the responsibility of preparing for the world of work as well as developing the social and emotional characteristics that will allow them to participate as contributing members of society.

It is often difficult for parents to help their retarded child achieve independence, and only few guides are available to parents of youngsters with Down Syndrome. There is a basic apprehension on many parents' part to have their child exposed to all the risks and responsibilities of growing up and becoming more independent. This is often tied with the concern that their child may be made fun of or taken advantage of. Not only parents, but all professionals tend to want to spare the adolescent with Down syndrome from being hurt or being placed in a potentially difficult situation. Yet, it is the overprotective behavior which in the long run may cause harm. The opportunities to experience risks, to make decisions, and to assume responsibility are essential to the development of internal control, self-confidence, and independence. Though one does not want the adolescent to fail or take continuous risks, there are occasions when he can learn through failure. Parents and professionals both have to recognize that an essential part of growing up is learning through experience. For the youngster with Down Syndrome this experience may at times be structured. However, it is important that there is an opportunity for him to make decisions, initiate actions and assume some of the responsibility of those actions if independence is to be achieved.

One factor hindering the adolescent with Down Syndrome in becoming more independent is the often observed tendency of parents and society to look upon this individual as an eternal child. Many people refer to young retarded adults as children and treat them as such. In the face of such perceptions, it is difficult to establish the necessary parental behaviors that will encourage the development of independence and responsibility.

Unlike other teenagers, the retarded adolescent gets very little help from his peers in his struggle for independence. He has infrequent relationships with other adolescents except in the school and few opportunities are available to meet with peers in unstructured recreational settings and during leisure time activities.

The school as well as the home will have to provide information to the adolescent with Down Syndrome about sex differences and sex roles in life. When children grow into adolescence, they have to understand the physical and social changes that take place during this particular time period in life. From the very beginning children need healthy and wholesome attitudes both about their own bodies and the functions of these bodies.

The amount of information and how it is given to an adolescent with Down Syndrome may differ from that of a nonhandicapped peer. Repetition and the use of direct and simple words are necessary. A retarded person is less able to guess, to fill in, or interpret from analysis. As a result, information should be given in a very concrete fashion. Use of pictures, verbal explanations, and specific examples known to the adolescent will help in getting the message understood.

An important aspect of growing up and passing through adolescence concerns educating the young person in regard to the bodily changes that occur at this time in life. The body of an adolescent girl with Down Syndrome will follow the usual pattern of development for all girls. She will need helpful instructions on the meaning of menstruation and the proper care of herself during this time. Although her mental age may resemble that of a younger child, the adolescent girl with Down Syndrome could start to menstruate at an age when other girls begin to have their monthly period. She will need to be told about this before it happens to avoid unnecessary fears. Teaching a retarded child how to handle sanitary napkins during menstruation can be achieved using specific language and direct assistance until the task is learned. Positive verbal reinforcement will help. The instructional process is similar to that which is used in toilet training. Most girls who have managed toilet habits also will be able to take care of menstruation comfortably. The girls should know that menstruation is a part of becoming a woman and a normal event happening to all girls.

Masturbation or rubbing the genitals occurs with retarded children just as it does with other children, although parents often get more upset when they observe this in their retarded child. If masturbation is observed too frequently or in public, one might have to find out why the child is doing this, and it might require some special attention. The adolescent might be bored or may not be getting any satisfaction from other activities. It may be that he or she does not get much fun out of life or his social environment is not treating him appropriately. One has to look then for a change in the environment. Masturbation does not have any more special meaning to the retarded than it has to the nonretarded person. Therefore, one should not get overly anxious, fearful, or even punish such behavior. When adults can react wisely and confidently, letting the child know that it is all right if he handles his genitals, then problems will usually not emerge. However, if one shames youngsters or fills them with fears, this may leave problems of both an immediate and long term nature.

Touching one's body should not be considered an unhealthy act but rather an appropriate response to the physiological changes which are occurring. Emphasis should be placed not upon eliminating such behaviors, but making sure that they are done in a socially acceptable fashion and not to the point that it is an obsession.

16 ═══

VOCATIONAL TRAINING

Siegfried M. Pueschel

Although it often involves considerable frustration and anxiety, parents will have to help the young adult with Down Syndrome move from the sheltered environment of the home into the world of work and toward forming relationships with nonretarded adults.

During the formative years of vocational development there is a need to have the young adult begin to experience in a very concrete fashion the essential components of career development. Through a process of experiencing different vocational opportunities, the young adult with Down Syndrome can begin to formulate vocational expectations. In addition to the process of identifying specific likes and dislikes, a prevocational program will provide an opportunity for the young adult to begin to accept responsibility for his or her actions and thus begin to share in the planning process for the future. It is important to have the person with Down Syndrome attempt to play a more active role in the decisionmaking process regarding his employment and his future.

Prior to becoming involved in vocational activities, the person with Down Syndrome should begin to be exposed to prevocational training activities. Initially, each student should be carefully evaluated with respect to ability, interest, and social skills. There should also be an opportunity for the student to test himself in many types of vocational activities. Through such an assessment process, it will be possible to develop an exploratory prevocational program.

In a work-study program, the student may spend a portion of his day in the classroom, increasing his academic skills. During the remainder of the day, the student may leave the school for an on-the-job training program in the community. Such a program may utilize the resources of a sheltered workshop or, in some cases, it may be a competitive employment situation in industry. The kind of placement will depend on the student's aptitude, ability, and readiness. The nature of the work experience will vary somewhat according to the design and philosophy of each particular program. Some programs begin the experience by immediately placing the student in the community.

The primary purpose of the work experience, however, is not to develop specific vocational skills, but rather to enable a student to attain good work habits and the interpersonal skills necessary to maintain a job. If in the course of training specific skills are acquired, they will be helpful in obtaining specific jobs later. Specific skill competencies should not be emphasized, however, at the expense of the effective dimensions of vocational behavior and adjustment to work.

Cooperation between the public school, the vocational rehabilitation agency, and the sheltered workshop is a prerequisite for developing a good program for the student with Down Syndrome. A work-study program should include a close working relationship between the public school teacher and the workshop staff so that academic programs may be made meaningful in terms of the young person's experience in the work program. Emphasis on special academic training, attitudes, patterns of behavior, and relationships with coworkers and supervisors should receive the attention of both the school and the workshop to assure maximum progress.

Based on an evaluation of his prevocational experience, parents and school will be able to decide together with the student which vocational training program will be of the greatest benefit. Once his abilities and skills have been determined, one can then recommend work in a sheltered workshop, an on-the-job training facility, or a training program within a vocational school. Various types of training in those settings can be utilized to develop an individual's potential for vocational adjustment.

A vocational training program for young persons with Down Syndrome should be designed to provide them with a structured and realistic vocational experience that will enable the student to achieve maximum success in either community employment or a sheltered workshop situation. This program must be based on the ultimate vocational needs of the student and should also emphasize the development of interpersonal skills required in most jobs. Success of the individual with Down Syndrome in the job market is in part based on his efficiency in doing a job, coupled with such character traits as steadiness, reliability, diligence, responsibility, and trustworthiness on the job. A person's social adjustment and his relationship with coworkers are frequently an important factor in attaining success on the job.

Most training programs are of limited duration, which unfortunately often leaves the student "half-trained." Because the limited funds of training programs are often terminated too early, no meaningful results can be achieved and the person with Down Syndrome loses the benefit of the investment that has been made. Therefore, a job training program should have built-in time flexibility and should take into consideration the student's progress and skill developments. A vocational training program should also have an associated placement program so that students once trained will be able to move into an appropriate working relationship.

Once on the job, an employee with Down Syndrome will need to establish a meaningful relationship with his employer and coworkers. Many job-trained persons with Down Syndrome are capable of carrying out job responsibilities. They often impress their employers with skills and attitudes that they were not able to verbalize when initially seeking employment. Many individuals who had previously been considered unemployable have been trained for employment and have found jobs. Others will be able to perform well in a sheltered work environment where there is less pressure placed upon production. The ultimate goal of all work programs is to prepare the young person to function at the highest level possible in employment—be it competitive or sheltered.

Undoubtedly, the first few days and weeks of adjustment on the job are critical. In some instances, frustrations faced in the new environment, coupled with an occasional traumatic experience that a new employee might encounter, could at times result in his losing his job after substantial investments have been made in training and placement. Therefore, during this initial adjustment assistance is needed to guide the young person with Down Syndrome in order to avoid failure and to prevent a premature withdrawal from a situation.

Too frequently, handicapped individuals, and in particular persons with Down Syndrome, are still vocationally stereotyped. They are often ushered into positions such as dishwashers and janitors. While these occupations might be complex and might be personally satisfying and rewarding to many individuals, they often represent a lack of consideration for the individual worker's interest and aptitude. Creativity and imagination can open up a wider variety of occupations for the handicapped person.

On the other hand, some retarded individuals might set vocational goals for themselves which cannot be realized. On occasion, parents also have inappropriate expectations for the student. Often these vocational aspirations carry with them educational requirements beyond the capabilities of the student. Teachers and counselors must help both students and parents establish realistic vocational choices which are functional and still satisfying to the individual.

Sometimes parents think that a low-paying job or an unskilled job is demeaning for their youngster. As a result, they deprive their son or daughter of an important working experience and an opportunity to develop greater interpersonal skills. Unfortunately, retarded youngsters are too often asked to do all the "dirty work." Situations where the individual with Down Syndrome may be misused should, of course, be avoided. He should be accepted for what he is and for what he can do, and be praised and paid accordingly.

Whether his employment is in private industry or in a sheltered workshop, a person with Down Syndrome will gain a feeling of self-worth and of making a contribution to the community. This experience is important for every person, but in particular for the handicapped individual. He should be given the opportunity to prove to himself and others that he is capable of doing things. Such an accomplishment will increase his self-esteem and satisfy his family. Society, too, should acknowledge his contribution.

In addition to the work aspect, vocational rehabilitation should focus on recreation and social adjustment. Adult recreational activities should be made available. The development of social adjustment skills will make it possible for the person with Down Syndrome to establish interpersonal relationships with others of similar interests. A person with Down Syndrome should be able to have the normal experiences of making friends. Parents, schools, and vocational centers can help in the development of interpersonal relationships by providing both individual and group counseling, along with ample opportunities to meet and get to know other people. With the proper use of vocational rehabilitation and recreation, and the development of social adjustment, the life of the person with Down Syndrome can become meaningful to himself and his parents. They will be better able to carry the responsibility of either keeping him at home or providing a group home. The resulting ongoing, warm, human relationships which are important for every human being will also give the person with Down Syndrome satisfaction and assist him in his pursuit of happiness.

17

PARTING FROM HOME

Siegfried M. Pueschel

In previous chapters we have stressed that opportunities and assistance should be provided for the child and adolescent with Down Syndrome to enable him to become as independent as possible. We have emphasized that independence training starts in infancy, that the early years are of the utmost importance in paving the way for the future, that during the school years social behaviors are shaped, and that the individual with Down Syndrome needs exposure to life experiences that will enable him to function optimally in society.

Now, on the threshold of his or her entry into adulthood new questions arise: How will the person with Down Syndrome use his acquired skills in the years ahead? How will he function in the community? And for parents, perhaps the most crucial question of all: What will become of him after we are gone?

If we have succeeded in giving our children the tools to accomplish things in life by inducing in them the desire to be curious and learn, if we have helped them develop ways to communicate, made them aware of their abilities, we will have opened up the avenue on which they will march into the future. If the youngsters have been trained in social graces, if undesirable habits have been avoided because of the teaching of acceptable social behaviors, if we have instilled in them the belief of self-worth, we shall have made a significant impact upon their future lives.

Current interest in mentally retarded persons has focused primarily on programs for young retarded children including children with Down Syndrome. There has been little emphasis on the retarded adult. Yet, there is a growing concern, especially for those retarded individuals who live in the community, to provide them with appropriate jobs, recreation, and social interactions.

The individual with Down Syndrome who has finished school and job training may leave home just like our other children to form new living arrangements. In planning community living for the adult with Down Syndrome, one has to define the individual needs of the person and then see whether the community is able to meet these needs. Like the rest of us, he will have both physiological and psychological needs. Physiological needs include those which must be satisfied if the person is to survive, such as food, clothing, and shelter. His bodily needs do not appear to differ significantly from those of the general population. The psychosocial needs of each individual may vary from culture to culture and person to person, but would include feelings of security, a sense of adequacy, and a need to love and to be loved. In addition, the adult with Down Syndrome has a need for appropriate counseling, recreational facilities, and work opportunities. Failure to satisfy these needs may lead to failure in community living. It is important that one considers these physiological and psychosocial needs since adults with Down Syndrome have often been treated as though their only problem were mental retardation. Experience has shown that the adult with Down Syndrome living in the community needs to be provided with services that are broad and comprehensive, as well as highly specific, if his needs are to be met at all.

The goals of a community program should provide conditions and circumstances to enable an adult person with Down Syndrome to adequately perform the activities of daily living, to live harmoniously in the community, to achieve the maximum level of economic productivity, and to fulfill normal civic responsibilities according to his abilities. Comprehensive personal, social, and vocational services should be provided in association with counseling, for both the person with Down Syndrome and his parents. These kinds of services should be coordinated with vocational preparation, job placement, and productive activity in a sheltered workshop or supervised employment. Recreational and leisure time activities should be included. Finally, we have to search for novel ways to make the life of the adult with Down Syndrome more meaningful.

There is also a need for educational programs for the community regarding the needs of the mentally retarded adult. We have to forget attitudes in society so that our young handicapped people will be accepted so that they may, to the best of their abilities, realistically participate in community life.

Planning for the person with Down Syndrome must be related to the community planning for all citizens, but especially for all handicapped persons. Coordination of various community services should be forthcoming so that adults with Down Syndrome will be provided with appropriate services. Planning for the adult with Down Syndrome in the community should involve those who receive services as well as those who provide them. When total responsibility for program planning and implementation rests with a particular agency, with little or no participation by the users of services, many misconceptions may be introduced. While some adults with Down Syndrome may indeed contribute in planning and implementing programs, others might be passive observers or unrealistically make suggestions which are not feasible or practical. As adults with Down Syndrome develop in maturity and social competence, they may well demonstrate capabilities for planning and self-directions in programs and decisionmaking that could contribute to their own independent living in the community.

In considering living arrangements for the adult with Down Syndrome, one should take into consideration such factors as age, sex, degree of mental handicap, medical and emotional problems, and job arrangements. It is important that living quarters not only be designed in terms of bed space, but take into account the total needs of the handicapped person. There may be homes where adults with Down Syndrome live in total independence. There may be others where parents or responsible relatives are in charge, or half-way house situations where considerable supervision and supportive services are available.

Epilogue

We all hope that in the future, instead of lip service, adults with Down Syndrome will be offered a status that observes their rights and privileges as citizens in a democratic society and, in a very real sense, preserves their human dignity. Society has to realize that the mentally retarded persons, including individuals with Down Syndrome, are people in their own right, in spite of their limited capacity for academic achievement. They have needs, wishes, and hopes which ought to be recognized. Instead of custodial supervision, novel programs should provide guidance and assistance to help the persons with Down Syndrome develop their own identities and lead their own lives as much as possible. Such optimism regarding the future will only come true if we retain a solid grip on the reality of the present and pass on the wisdom derived from the past.

Bibliography

Barnard, Kathryn E., and Powell, Marcene, Jr. *Teaching the Mentally Retarded Child*. St. Louis: Mosby, 1972.

Blamenfeld, Thompson and Vogel, eds. *Help Them Grow*. Nashville: Abingdon Press, 1971.

Brightman, Alan. *Like Me*. Cambridge, Mass.: Harvard University, Behavioral Educational Projects, Inc., 1975.

Brinkworth, Rex. *The Unfinished Child: Early Treatment and Training for the Infant with Down's Syndrome*. Royal Society of Health 2: 73, 1975.

Brinkworth, Rex, and Collens, Joseph. *Improving Mongol Babies*. Belfast, Northern Ireland: Melbourne Observer Press, 1969.

Canning, Claire and Joseph. *The Gift of Martha*. Boston, Mass.: Resource Development/Children's Hospital Medical Center, 1975.

Carlson, Bernice Wells, and Ginglend, David R., eds. *Play Activities for the Retarded Child*. Nashville: Abingdon Press, 1961.

Cowie, Valerie A. *A Study of the Early Development of Mongols*. New York/London: Pergamon Press, 1966.

Cunningham, C.C., and Sloper, P. *Parents of Down's Syndrome Babies: Their Early Needs*. Working paper—Hester Adrian Research Center, University of Manchester.

de Vries-Kruyt, T. *A Special Gift: The Story of Jan*. New York: Peter H. Wyden, 1966.

Dittman, Laura. *The Mentally Retarded Child At Home*. U.S. Department of H.E.W., Washington, D.C.: Children's Bureau Publication, 1966.

Doorly, Ruth. *Our Jimmy.* Norwood, Mass.: Service Associates, 1967.

Hayden, Alice. Down Syndrome Children at the University of Washington, *Intervention Strategies for Risk Infants and Young Children.* Baltimore: University Park Press, 1974.

Horrobin, J. Margaret, and Rynders, John E. *To Give an Edge.* Minneapolis: Colwell Press, 1974.

Hunt, Nigel. *The World of Nigel Hunt: The Diary of a Mongoloid Youth.* New York: Taplinger Publishing Company, 1967.

Koch, Richard and de la Cruz, Felix F. *Down's Syndrome (Mongolism).* New York: Brunner/Mazel, 1975.

Koch, Richard and Kathryn Jean. *Understanding the Mentally Retarded Child: A New Approach.* New York: Random House, 1975.

Mentally Handicapped Children: A Handbook for Parents and Your Mongol Baby. London: National Association for Mental Health, 1968.

Perske, Robert and Martha. *New Directions for Parents of Persons Who Are Retarded.* Nashville: Abingdon Press, 1973.

Pitt, David. *Your Down's Syndrome Child.* Arlington, Texas: National Association for Retarded Citizens, 1974.

Roberts, Nancy and Bruce. *David.* Richmond, Virginia: John Knox Press, 1968.

Roberts, Nancy and Bruce. *You and Your Retarded Child.* St. Louis: Concordia Publishing House, 1974.

Smith, David W., and Wilson, Ann Asper. *The Child with Down's Syndrome (Mongolism).* Philadelphia: W.B. Saunders, 1973.

Toward Independent Feeding: The Young Child With Down's Syndrome. New England Developmental Disabilities Communication Center, 1973.

PERIODICALS

Closer Look
P.O. Box 492, Washington, D.C. 20013
Mental Retardation News
National Association for Retarded Citizens, P.O. Box 6109, Arlington, Texas 76011
The Exceptional Parent
Psy-Ed Corporation, Room 708 Statler Office Building, 20 Providence Street, Boston, Massachusetts 02116
Sharing Our Caring
M. Bridge Chlidren's Hospital, P.O. Box 196, Milton, Washington 98354.
Down's Syndrome News
P.O. Box 400, Milton, Washington 98354

ABOUT THE AUTHORS

Siegfried M. Pueschel, M.D., M.P.H., is the director of the Child Development Center at Rhode Island Hospital and Associate Professor in Pediatrics at the Brown University Program in Medicine. For six years he was the director of the Down Syndrome Program at Children's Hospital Medical Center in Boston.

Claire D. Canning received her bachelor's degree from Newton College of the Sacred Heart and continues to study in special education. She is the mother of five children. Because the birth of their last child with Down Syndrome was such a traumatic experience, she spends much of her time trying to ease the shock of this experience for others. She is the author of *The Gift of Martha* and many other magazine articles emphasizing the positive aspects of mental retardation. She is a frequent speaker and is active in community work for the handicapped.

Ann Murphy, M.S.W., is presently the Director of Social Work for the Developmental Evaluation Clinic at Children's Hospital Medical Center in Boston.

Elizabeth Zausmer, M.Ed., R.P.T., is the director of training in physical therapy at the Developmental Evaluation Clinic at Children's Hospital Medical Center in Boston. She is an adjunct assistant professor at Boston University's Sargent College of Allied Health Professions and a lecturer at Simmons College in Boston.